water

The Foundation of Youth, Health, and Beauty

IMPAKT|health

water

The Foundation of Youth, Health, and Beauty

by
William D. Holloway, Jr.,
and Herb Joiner-Bey, ND

Published by:
IMPAKT Health
2551 31st St.
Boulder, CO 80301
E-mail: info@impakt.com
Fax: 303-440-7446
www.impakt.com

The information in this book is for educational purposes only and is derived from a judicious synthesis of traditional and clinical experience and verified by scientific principles and research. It is intended for use by professionals seeking to apply the principles of natural medicine to the needs of their patients and by patients under the direct supervision and guidance of such professionals.

The authors do not intend to suggest that people should self-diagnose and/or self-medicate without the sound judgment and seasoned counsel of a well-informed healthcare provider. We strongly urge the patient to consult an appropriately educated practitioner before making any changes to health maintenance or therapeutic regimens.

I would like to first thank my coauthor Dr. Herb Joiner-Bey for his tireless research and skills that have made this book a reality. His understanding of the human body and all its functions provided the foundation of understanding that helps convey the critical importance of water and hydration for the human body. His willingness to search for the truth in nature and remain open minded sets him apart from those who accept past doctrine without challenge.

Second, I would like to thank Penta™ water customers, many of whom have written or called me personally to express their experience with Penta™ water. Their encouragement and belief in our product makes our hard work much more rewarding.

Third, I would like to thank the natural health stores and health-care practitioners who carry and recommend Penta™ water. Thanks to them, Penta™ water is available throughout the United States, and internationally through our agents in the United Kingdom, Hong Kong, Australia, and New Zealand.

Fourth, I would like to thank our sales representatives and the entire staff of Bio-Hydration Research Lab, Inc. They have embraced our mission and helped make our water available across the United States in a short period of time.

Finally, I would like to thank my wife, G. R. Holloway, for her unwavering support, understanding, and hard work. As an inventor, she is my greatest discovery—my love, soul mate, and best friend. And to my son, Michael Holloway, thanks for his brilliance, hard work, and support. It makes every day we work together a pleasure. Also to my son, Chad Holloway, who gave his time and energies to make our dreams a reality.

William D. Holloway, Jr.

First, I must acknowledge the breakthrough inventiveness of Bill Holloway and his son, Michael, relative to stabilizing microclustered water without using chemicals. Engineers are those who take the theories and discoveries of scientists and apply them for human benefit in the everyday world. Bill and Michael have made a great contribution to the wellness of humanity. Those of us in the field of natural medicine have known about the benefits of adequate hydration for ages, but Bill's influence has taken my appreciation for water's place in human health to a whole new level of understanding.

Second, I acknowledge Dr. Fereydoon Batmanghelidj, the heroic Iranian medical doctor who discovered the wide-ranging healing properties of water while under the threat of execution by the revolutionary government of his native land. Since the time of his incarceration as a political prisoner, attending to the health needs of other prisoners with the healing power of water, he has taken a courageous stand over the last 20 years for that which is simple and effective in healing and readily available to all people everywhere.

Third, I acknowledge G. R. Holloway, Hoppy Rodenbaugh, and Jack Barrient, whose contributions to this project have been invaluable.

Fourth, I acknowledge Karolyn Gazella of IMPAKT Health (a division of InnerDoorway, LLC) whose professionalism and grace as an editor and publisher are an author's wish come true.

Herb Joiner-Bey, ND

water

The Foundation of Youth, Health, and Beauty

table of contents

introduction
A New Look at an Old Friend

The subject of water might seem bland and mundane, but water is one of the most powerful healing and life-giving substances. For scientists, the presence of this substance determines the ability of a planet in our universe to sustain life as we know it. We use water every day to drink, cook, bathe, clean, and play. It always seems to be there when we need it—if we are lucky. A thirsty Bedouin tribesman far from an oasis would not regard water so casually. He might even kill for it to save his parched children.

In Taoism, the single major spiritual philosophy indigenous to China, sages encourage us to know the Absolute (the Creator of the Universe) by observing its creation: nature. Regrettably, history shows that humanity's observational skills have often lacked insight. We take for granted so much that is precious. We may note the wild flowers in the field, but we have little appreciation for the moist, nutrient-rich soil that allows them to flourish. We look, but we do not see. We see, but we do not observe. We observe, but we do not

> "What we observe is not nature itself, but nature exposed to our method of questioning."
>
> —Werner Heisenberg, physicist

1

realize. We realize, but we do not act accordingly. Thus the suffering of humanity is needlessly perpetuated.

In our zeal to amass the material comforts afforded by Western industrialization, we have put tremendous toxic strain on the natural living environment that sustains our lives. This disregard for our own long-term well-being is exemplified in the modern world by the pollution of the most basic substance we put into our bodies—water—as well as modern conventional medicine's disregard for its potential to heal and prevent disease.

For the educationally conditioned intellect, eager for esoteric answers to complex problems, it seems too simplistic to believe that something as innocuous as water could have therapeutic potential. But this commonly held view is based on misinformation, lack of pertinent clinical experience, and a prejudicial unwillingness to abandon old views in favor of more enlightened understanding.

At the grassroots level, however, and among some progressive scientists and healing practitioners, views about water are changing. An undeniable accumulation of evidence is forcing open-minded people to regard with clearer vision the true value and utility of one of the dearest friends to human health.

It is the fervent hope of the authors that this book, a general overview of what is now understood about the way in which pure water benefits human health, will lay a foundation for discussion, healing modalities, and future research on this underappreciated necessity of life.

chapter one
Living Water: The Human Body

Water is the most basic chemical constituent of all living things, from protozoa to sperm whales and phytoplankton to sequoias. In fact, it can be said that all physical life forms on Earth consist of water that is compartmentalized into basic units of life, called "cells."

Water is the predominant compound in the human body. Every nook and cranny not occupied by proteins (e.g., structural members, enzymes, antibodies), fats (e.g., cell membranes, fat deposits in fat cells), carbohydrates (e.g., glycogen, chondroitin sulfate), or bone components (e.g., hydroxyapitite crystals), is occupied by water molecules. The omnipresence of water throughout the body gives it powerful local and systemic influence over everything that happens within human beings to sustain life.

At birth, the body of a full-term baby is 78 percent water. As we age, that percentage declines to 72 percent of fat-free body weight for normal young adults and 50 percent among the elderly.

The brain consists of 85 percent water. The water content of muscle tissue is 75 percent, 10 percent for fat tissue, and even bone tissue is 22 percent water.

For a 150-pound young adult male, the 72 percent water content amounts to 45 quarts, 30 of which are located within cells (intracellular) and 15 of which are located outside of cells (extracellular). These figures are a little lower in women. The ratio of intracellular to extracellular water is approximately two to one in healthy young adults. Of the 15 quarts of extracellular water, three are composed of plasma of the blood, and other smaller quantities constitute the lymph fluid within tissues, the cerebrospinal fluid, the vitreous humor fluid of the eye, the secretions of the respiratory and intestinal mucous membranes, the synovial fluid that lubricates the joints, and other fluid compartments of the body. (Garrow)

The body uses all this water as the base for many biochemical functions. For example, evidence suggests that the nervous system uses water to carry brain neurotransmitters through microstream waterways along nerves to reach the periphery of the body. (Batmanghelidj)

Leaks in the Water Bag

Throughout the day, water escapes from the body through perspiration, urine, feces, tears, nasal discharges, respiratory exhaled moisture, and other pathways. Losses are increased by the consumption of the natural diuretics caffeine, theophylline, and theobromine in beverages like coffee, black and green tea, and soft drinks. It is estimated that we lose nine to 12 cups of water on a cool day even without exercising. (Bird) For optimal health, these losses must be replaced by adequate ingestion of water sources in beverages and food. Food is an important consideration, because it contains water, and water is generated during food metabolism. (Berne)

Controlling the Floodgates

According to the current principles of physiology, the control of overall water balance in the body resides with the hypothalamus, the structure at the base of the brain that also controls the endocrine hormonal system. Osmoreceptor cells in the hypothalamus detect the concentration of substances, such as sodium chloride, dissolved in the blood. If the concentration of solutes (dissolved substances) gets too high, the osmoreceptors signal other hypothalamus cells to form antidiuretic hormone (ADH), also called vasopressin.

Antidiuretic hormone is stored in the posterior portion of the pituitary gland. When it is released into the bloodstream, it stimulates the collecting ducts of the kidney filtration units to become permeable to water; that is, the ducts allow water in the filtered fluid to pass through them before it exits the kidney via urine. The water leaves the filtered urine in the collecting ducts and returns to the bloodstream. This process restores normal concentration of solutes in those fluids and reduces the amount of water in the urine, making it more concentrated. Every normal human being has a set point of body fluid solute concentration at which ADH release is triggered. The release of ADH also is triggered by significant decreases in blood volume and blood pressure. This response is important to maintain adequate flow of blood to the heart, brain, and other vital organs. (Berne)

Quenching Thirst

Cells in the thirst center of the hypothalamus control the sensation of thirst and are distinct from osmoreceptors. Interestingly, both thirst cells and osmoreceptors are sensitive to only certain solutes in body fluids, such as sodium, and are relatively insensitive to other solutes, such as urea. (Berne) Even small amounts of fluid intake quickly satisfy the sensation of thirst before water leaves the gastrointestinal tract to dilute solutes in blood plasma. This is the result of receptors in the mouth, throat, and upper portion of the gastrointestinal tract. However, the effect of these local receptors is short in duration. Thirst returns quickly until the concentration of solutes in the plasma is restored to the set point that signals satisfaction for the thirst center. (Berne)

Unfortunately, the sensitivity of the thirst center declines with age. Consequently, it is common for the elderly to succumb to physical collapse resulting from dehydration if they are not vigilant in hydrating themselves adequately throughout the day. In addition, thirst is not a good indicator of the need for water in infants and children, patients suffering from a host of illnesses, or athletes and laborers engaged in strenuous physical activity. (Bird, Short)

Blood, Sweat, and Tears

Optimal physical health requires optimal functioning of each cell in the body in harmonious relationship with all other cells. Optimal functioning of each cell requires ideal cell hydration.

We tend to take our bodily functions for granted until something goes seriously wrong. Unless we live in a water-scarce region, water is at the bottom of the barrel of our conscious personal attention and priorities. However, consider the body's physiological priorities regarding the water necessary to maintain itself in its environment. The following are body fluids that rely on an adequate water supply.

— Blood, which supplies all cells with oxygen and nutrients and provides a means of disposing waste materials
— Lymph fluids, which wash undesirable microbes and debris away from extracellular regions
— Digestive secretions of the salivary glands, stomach, small intestine, pancreas, liver, and colon

— Urine for the excretion of water-soluble waste materials

— Cerebrospinal fluid of the central nervous system

— Fluid transport channels of the peripheral nervous system

— Lubricating fluids between the serosal membranes separating the heart from the pericardial sac, the lungs from the inner wall of the chest, and the abdominal organs from the inner wall of the abdominal cavity

— Lubricating fluids secreted by the synovial membranes of the joints

— Vaginal secretions and menstrual discharges

— Semen (i.e., secretions of prostate gland and seminal vesicles)

— Mucous secretions of the nose, throat, bronchial tubes, and lungs

— Perspiration and water that evaporates from the skin to regulate body temperature

— Tears

— Fluids of the vitreous humor of the eye

— Water that cushions shock by surrounding the water-attracting biochemical constituents of the vertebral disks and joint cartilage

— Water that surrounds structural constituents of connective tissue

Ninety percent of the interior constituents of every cell in the body are water molecules. To get a feeling for the quantities of water-based fluid secretions the body generates daily, let's take a closer look at the gastrointestinal tract. The daily quantities of output are amazing: 1,000 ml = 1 liter or approximately 1 quart. The following is a breakdown of gastrointestinal secretions. (Berne)

— Saliva: 1,500 ml

— Gastric secretions: 2,000 ml

— Bile from the liver: 500 ml

— Intestinal secretions: 1,200 ml

— Fecal excretion: 100 ml

A tremendous amount of the water in these secretions is absorbed by the small intestine and colon. Nevertheless, these secretions are made from water extracted from the blood and secretory cells. If optimal water supplies are lacking, gastrointestinal function is impaired. This is only one example of the negative effects dehydration can have on one organ system. The fact is dehydration inhibits every one of the body's organs in ways we are just beginning to recognize. It is no wonder the body puts an extremely high priority on adequate water intake, despite the tendency of many people to ignore or circumvent this need.

Signs and Symptoms of Dehydration

Dehydration is a serious medical condition that must not be taken lightly. It must be resolved quickly and efficiently to prevent dire medical consequences. The symptoms of dehydration include

— fatigue and weakness;

— headaches;

— rough, dry skin;

— dry mucous membranes in nose, mouth, or throat;

— nosebleeds (especially in dry interior air during winter);

— dark, concentrated, strong-smelling urine in small quantities;

— irritability;

— irrational behavior;

— constipation;

— nausea;

— intestinal cramps;

— weak, irregular pulse;

— low blood pressure; and

— shallow, rapid breathing.

Women are at greater risk for dehydration, because they have less muscle mass and lower body water content than men. (Bird) In later chapters, we will explore in detail the medical consequences of dehydration and disease states that can be dramatically improved by simply drinking pure water.

Dying by Drying

In the long run, ignorance is not bliss. What people don't know is killing them. It has been estimated that almost half the American population unknowingly suffers from some degree of dehydration. One third of Americans drink three or fewer servings of water daily. Many people suffer from what Michael Lam, MD, calls "sub-clinical dehydration." A three percent loss in body water volume causes fatigue and organ dysfunction. A 10 percent loss can be life threatening. By the time people experience a dry mouth, the body has already begun to suffer the effects of dehydration. Dry mouth is a late-stage manifestation of water need in many people. (Lam)

First Things First: Listening to the Body's Real Nutritional Priorities

In nutritional science, substances ingested to support the functioning of the body are divided into major groups: micronutrients and macronutrients. Micronutrients are vitamins, minerals, and accessory food factors. Macronutrients are divided into the well-known categories of protein, fats, and carbohydrates. Unfortunately, because pure water provides no caloric potential, it has been excluded from categorization as a macronutrient. To put this oversight in perspective, consider that a person can survive for weeks without ingesting any of the macronutrients or micronutrients listed above, but only a few days without water. For human survival, water is definitely the most important nutrient, and for optimal health, it is the most undervalued part of the human diet. Water is also the most underused tool in healing, even among many practitioners of natural medicine. We will provide a more detailed discussion of water's healing potential in later chapters.

How Much Water is Enough?

Water intake requirements vary according to individual needs and circumstances. Under ordinary conditions, an average individual living in an environment with moderate temperature and humidity requires about eight to 10 cups of water daily. (Short) If you wish to be more precise, take the number of pounds you weigh and divide that number in half. The result is the number of fluid ounces of pure water that you should drink each day. For example, a 200-pound person should drink 100 fluid ounces (about 12 eight-ounce glasses) of pure water daily. Notice that we wrote "water," not "fluids." The reason for this distinction will be made clear when we discuss cellular hydration and how to optimize it. These water intake recommendations are in addition to any other beverages.

Hot, Cold, or Tepid

People are in the habit of drinking fluids, including water, at varying temperatures. Does the temperature of foods and beverages have any effect on how the body functions? According to the principles of Traditional Chinese Medicine, it does. The principles of

Western physiology may lend some credence to this idea, as well. According to some authorities in Chinese medicine, the consumption of cold food and drink is a hindrance to optimal health and wellness among people in Western civilization.

The average person knows that the normal oral temperature for a human being is approximately 98.6 degrees Fahrenheit. The internal temperature of the body, however, is higher. For example, the interior temperature of the heart is approximately 106 degrees. These warm temperatures are needed for the optimal functioning of biochemical processes that sustain life. The ingestion of large amounts of cold food and beverages tends to inhibit these processes. This is particularly true of the functioning of the upper regions of the gastrointestinal tract, particularly the stomach. The stomach cannot fulfill its digestive function efficiently if its tissue temperature is lowered by cold food and drink. This phenomenon contributes to indigestion. Full functioning cannot return until the food in the stomach and stomach tissues rise to normal interior body temperature. The colder the food and beverages and the larger the quantity consumed, the longer it takes the stomach to reach optimal functioning temperature. For this reason, it is prudent to limit the amount of cold food and beverages consumed daily. In particular, since we are recommending the ingestion of large quantities of pure water, we also recommend that this water be at room temperature or warmer to minimize inhibition of efficient digestive function.

Special Needs for Special People

Particular care must be taken to adequately hydrate people who, because of special circumstances, may have need for an even greater intake of water. These people include

— infants fed high-protein formulas (be careful not to over-hydrate infants);
— patients suffering from disorders whose symptoms include fever, vomiting, diarrhea, respiratory discharges, and other avenues of water loss;
— patients taking diuretic medicines;
— people eating high-protein diets;
— people living in environments with high atmospheric temperatures; and
— people engaged in strenuous physical activity, such as athletes and physical laborers. (Short)

chapter two
Working Water: The Cell in Action

Trickle Down: Theory and Reality

The life of a multicellular organism depends on the meticulously organized and smoothly coordinated efforts of all cells within the organism. Biochemistry, as modern science understands it, occurs at the cellular level. Wellness of the whole person depends on the biochemical and energetic well-being of every cell in the body. And the well-being of each cell depends on how well its nutritional, biochemical, and energetic needs are met.

The human body is essentially a watery, living tube arising from the three tissue layers of the embryo. The ectoderm layer produces the skin (i.e., the outer surface of the tube) and the nervous system, from which nerves throughout the entire organism grow. The endoderm layer produces the gastrointestinal lining (i.e., the inner surface of the tube). The mesoderm produces all the major structures between these two surfaces, including muscle, bone, and organs. This watery, human body-tube is composed of 20 to 30 trillion cells, all derived from the fertilization of a single human egg cell. As daughters of the fertilized egg, they are members of the same biological family. With the exception of fat cells, every one of these trillions of cell siblings is 90 percent water. That means every cell contains billions of water molecules. The water in each cell is sequestered from the exterior by the dual-layered fatty acid cell membrane.

For a cell to be supplied with all the water it needs, the water a person drinks must overcome several obstacles to reach the inner parts of the cell. Water must be able to

— diffuse through the mucous membrane cells lining the gastrointestinal tract (i.e., the inner lining of the body tube),
— enter the general circulation of the bloodstream,
— diffuse through the capillary wall and surrounding connective tissue, and
— diffuse through the aquaporin protein water channels in the cell membrane.

At first glance, these obstacles seem easy to overcome. Water traverses these barriers throughout the day, every day of our lives. But this process involves far more than most people, including scientists and health professionals, even realize. For reasons that we will address through the remainder of this book, the optimal hydration of cells does not occur as efficiently and effortlessly as has been supposed since the beginning of the sciences of cell biology and physiology. Recent discoveries have shed new light on what is really required to hydrate the human body optimally at the cellular level. To begin to understand the requirements for cell hydration, let's take a closer look at some key features of this most basic unit of life.

Cell Anatomy

We will not attempt to discuss all the details of cell anatomy and biology. Instead, we will emphasize major structural characteristics that affect the influx of water and the behavior of water within the cell.

Water and oil do not mix. It is precisely this mutual exclusivity of water and oil that allows the miracle of life to exist. Each cell in the body is surrounded by a fatty membrane that keeps intracellular water in place and carefully selects which exterior substances, including extracellular water, are allowed to enter.

To cell biologists, the influence of the three membranes of the cell—the cell, nuclear, and mitochondrial (energy-generating power-house) membranes—is so great, many scientists believe that many diseases begin at the membrane level. The reason for this belief is clear. The membrane is the "skin" and "peripheral nervous system" of the cell, wielding powerful control over that which enters or leaves it. The membrane strongly influences how the cell responds to substances and entities in its environment, such as hormones, toxins, nutrients, waste, oxygen, carbon dioxide, water, microbes, and the immune system's white blood cells. Let's take an even closer look at this critical component of the cell.

Border Crossing

The cell membrane is made of a double layer of fatty acid molecules called phospholipids. Each phospholipid is made up of a three-carbon backbone called glycerol, to which are attached one phosphate group and two fatty acids derived from fats in the diet. Because the cell membrane is made of fatty (oily) substances, it is difficult for water or water-soluble solutes (dissolved sub-stances) to pass through it. However, protein channels in the membrane permit the entry of water and water-soluble materials. These protein channels, spanning the entire membrane, are called intrinsic membrane proteins. The membrane also contains proteins residing on its outer surface that serve other purposes. These are called "extrinsic membrane proteins." The cell membrane is, therefore, a "fluid mosaic" of phospholipids and proteins. (Berne) Until recently, the exact means by which water entered the cell had not been precisely identified. It was assumed that water simply passed through the membrane, because the membrane was somehow semipermeable. Then, in 1992, a Johns Hopkins researcher discovered protein water channels that he named "aquaporins."

Aquaporins

The ability to control water intake and release is fundamental to life. Aquaporin water channels provide this needed control.

Aquaporins constitute a large family of protein channels, which span cell membranes. They transport water across cell membranes so quickly that it is limited only by the rate of diffusion of water molecules (i.e., osmosis). At least ten distinct categories of aquaporins and at least 200 different forms exist. Aquaporins are found in a wide variety of organisms—humans, animals, bacteria, and plants.

Each aquaporin consists of six tilted helices plus two half-helices that dip into the membrane from outside and meet in the middle. Together they form a right-handed coil bundle. A single water pathway is formed in the center of the protein. On cell membranes, four aquaporin monomers (single units) connect into a tetramer (unit of four). The stability of this complex may arise from the contribution of each monomer as a tight-fitting wedge in the tetramer. Both ends of the chain of amino acids forming the protein components of aquaporins are found on the interior side of the cell membrane.

At its narrowest point, an aquaporin has a diameter of only three angstroms (one ten billionth of meter). A single water molecule has a diameter of 2.8 angstroms. Therefore, the size of the aquaporin opening is just large enough to allow the passage of water and oxygen molecules, but small enough to exclude larger ions and molecules. Laboratory experimentation on aquaporins has revealed that water influx is inhibited by the addition of mercury and other heavy metals. The structure of the aquaporin can explain this effect. A cysteine bonding unit projects into the pore and is the site of inhibition by mercury. When a heavy metal bonds to this cysteine unit, the pore is induced to close, terminating the flow of water through that channel. Other bonding sites are also crucial to the high degree of selectivity observed in aquaporins.

Filtering the Fluids

Through observation, researchers have concluded that the workings of aquaporins are nature's way of purifying water before it enters the cell. The passage of water is facilitated by the lightning-fast making and breaking of hydrogen bonds between water molecules and components of the aquaporins. The efficiency of this process of transport is astounding. Under ideal conditions, one aquaporin can accommodate the flow of three billion water molecules per second. In terms our minds can grasp more easily, an aquaporin-imbedded membrane measuring 10 by 10 centimeters can filter one liter of water in seven seconds. In effect, the aquaporin system is equipped to handle the flux of water molecules at the rate at which water naturally diffuses, without delaying flow. The efficiency of this system can easily meet the hydration needs of cells if it is not inhibited from performing its natural function. (Echevarria)

Aquaporins in Health and Disease

Aquaporins play critical roles in the function of many tissues and organs throughout the body. For example, the efficient functioning of aquaporins is essential to the performance of tissues in the lungs, kidneys, eyes, and capillary membranes throughout the body.

From our discussion of how the body prevents the dangerous loss of water by drawing water from the kidney collecting ducts into the bloodstream, it should be clear how important aquaporins are to kidney function. Many tissues, including lung airways and secretory glands, have complex patterns of multiple aquaporins. Aquaporins have been scientifically linked to a number of illnesses. Diabetes insipidus, which originates in the kidneys, may result from functional disruptive mutations in genes coding for kidney aquaporins. Genetic defects in the aquaporins of the lens of the eye can contribute to the development of cataracts.

Many disorders may produce secondary decreases or increases in aquaporin expression. Bipolar disorder (i.e., manic depression) is commonly treated with lithium, and increased urination is a side effect. Lithium causes a 90 percent decrease in kidney aquaporin expression. Patients with congestive heart failure often die from pulmonary edema (i.e., fluid infiltration in the lungs) caused by water retention. This problem occurs concurrently with increased aquaporin expression.

Structure in Action

Water is the most abundant substance in the body, with protein coming in second. Protein provides the major structural and functional components of the body and every cell within it. Every life process depends on this class of molecules. The range of protein's functions is immense and affects cell infrastructure, membrane transport, and the transport of fatty materials in the blood. In addition, many proteins serve as antibodies of the immune system as well as enzymes—the catalysts for all biochemical processes. Proteins are macromolecules—large chains of amino acids. In the field of architecture, the form of an edifice is designed to fit its intended function. And so it is with the structure of proteins. The function of a protein arises from its form—its three-dimensional shape. The unique sequence of the 20 amino acids coded by human deoxryibonucleic acid (DNA), "the genetic master compound," determines the shape or form of a protein. The unique sequence of a particular kind of protein is determined by the unique sequence of coding genes on the DNA of chromosomes that initiate the synthesis of that protein. (Champe, Garrow)

Waters of Architecture

Nothing in life happens in a vacuum. Context and environment are essential to the fulfillment of function, and proteins are no exception. The environment not only allows proteins to function as necessary, but also supports their endeavors. Water molecules provide that environment. In order to fulfill their respective missions, proteins must bend, twist, and contort their primary amino acid strands into secondary, tertiary, and quaternary forms. The hydrophobic (i.e., water-avoiding) and hydrophilic (i.e., water-attracting) interactions between water and protein strands drive the conformational changes needed for proteins to realize their ultimate functional form. In other words, the final shape of a protein is determined by the manner in which water and protein strands are attracted to or repelled by each other. As a lubricating agent, water facilitates the breaking and re-establishing of hydrogen bonds and other links between the various parts of protein. When the appropriate bonding is in place, water molecules are critical to the continued integrity and stability of protein structure. (Watterson, Chaplin) Because of the flexibility of the bonds among various portions of protein strands, large protein molecules have, under ideal conditions, the flexibility for dynamic action during rapid, life-sustaining biochemical interactions. This flexibility requires optimal hydration of protein molecules. (Watterson, Chaplin)

The internal architecture of the cell is composed of microtubules and microfilaments made of protein. Water, which has a reinforced, gel-like structure within the cell, serves as architectural reinforcement for the cell protein infrastructure. The dynamic, structural renovation of cells requires the unique contribution of water molecules every step of the way.

For these reasons, it is clear that proteins, the compounds that provide structure and biochemical function in the human body, are absolutely dependent on the full collaboration of water. Thus, optimal protein function demands ideal cell hydration.

Nuclear Waters

The heart of the cell, or nucleus, is surrounded by its own fatty-acid membrane. Within the boundary of the membrane lie the chromosomes composed of DNA. Molecules of messenger ribonucleic acid (mRNA) are also within the nucleus. Water molecules are intimately bound to both these compounds by hydrogen bonds in a manner that facilitates their critical functions. DNA carries the gene sequence codes, which are copied by mRNA and carried outside the nucleus to cell structures that use the codes to synthesize chains of amino acids (i.e., proteins). As the biochemical partners maintaining the structure and function of DNA and mRNA, water molecules are indispensable to the command and control activities of the cell. (Chaplin)

Upon deeper reflection, we discover that the role water plays in the unfolding of life is even more profound. The genetic code defines the structure of proteins by delineating unique sequences of amino acids. Water molecules drive the protein amino acid strands into their functional shapes and forms using hydrophobic and hydrophilic forces. It can, therefore, be concluded that the genetic coding sequences on the DNA molecule are arranged in a fashion that specifically anticipates the conformational interaction of water molecules required to finish the protein generating tasks. The process is somewhat like the construction of a building. Protein is the edifice, DNA is the architect, mRNA is the construction foreman, the ER and tRNA are skilled craftsmen, and water molecules are the laborers and maintenance workers. This interdependent interaction among DNA, mRNA, ER, tRNA, protein, and water defines a fundamental biochemical relationship that generates and sustains life.

Water Power: Hydrolysis

Another major role played by water within the cell is called hydrolysis, the biochemical process of adding water molecules to other molecules. These chemical reactions are paramount to the efficient functioning of each cell's life-sustaining activities. One of the most important chemical reactions involves the molecule that serves as the energy currency of every cell, adenosine triphosphate (ATP), and the molecule that serves as the energy reserve, creatine phosphate. These molecules are well-known by athletes, because they provide stamina for athletic performance. They also provide the energy for all daily activities.

Adenosine triphosphate is formed by sequentially adding three phosphate groups to the compound adenosine. Creatine phosphate, which exists mainly in muscle cells, is formed simply by adding a phosphate group to creatine. This process allows the two compounds to store energy derived from food in the form of high-energy chemical bonds linked to the phosphate groups. Enzymes catalyze these reactions, releasing water molecules into the cell.

When cells need to retrieve stored energy, the high-energy phosphate bonds must be broken by enzymes, adding water molecules to replace the disconnected phosphate groups. For this reason, the cell must be at optimal hydration to extract energy efficiently from ATP and creatine phosphate. Any water deficit within the cell will limit the availability of energy for cell functions and daily activities throughout the entire body. Body-wide cell dehydration is experienced as fatigue, loss of mental clarity and focus, and the inability to perform as desired.

Cell Hydration is Imperative

Optimal cell function demands optimal cell hydration. As the most abundant constituent of life on all levels, water is an intimate partner and participant in every biochemical reaction that occurs within every cell and tissue. We dare not neglect a substance that is so critical to our well-being.

chapter three
Dancing Water:
Dynamic Interplay of Molecules

What's So Special About H2O?

Like humans, every other living thing on Earth is composed mainly of water. As the basis for life, water is probably the most studied, yet least understood substance on the planet.

Consisting of two hydrogen atoms attached to an oxygen atom by covalent bonds, water is one of the simplest and smallest compounds in existence. Yet water's unusual properties and behavior are surprisingly complex and intriguing to scientists who have studied its mysteries.

Consider the three-dimensional structure of the water molecule. Imagine the oxygen atom at the center of a tetrahedron (the geometric figure that has identical, equal-sided triangles making up each of its four sides). The two hydrogen atoms are located at two of the four corners of the tetrahedron. The other two corners are unoccupied. This somewhat asymmetrical arrangement of atoms— reminiscent of a plump boomerang—generates all kinds of interesting interactions as water molecules do their liquid dance.

Based on this unique structural model, the dance is even more complex than one might expect. The hydrogen nuclei (protons) of a water molecule are not permanently bonded to the oxygen atom of that molecule. There is a tremendous amount of proton exchange among water molecules. The rate of exchange is so fast that scientists treat the triad of atoms in each molecule as a stable relationship.

The Ties That Bind

One of the primary ways water molecules in the liquid state relate to each other is called "hydrogen bonding." This phenomenon occurs because the oxygen atom in each molecule is greedy about holding onto the electrons from the two hydrogen atoms, and the hydrogens comply without giving up the electrons completely. Consequently, the electrons spend more time around the oxygen atom than the hydrogen nuclei. This tendency places a slight negative charge on the oxygen side of the molecule, and a slight positive charge on each of the hydrogens. The positive charges on the hydrogens are electromagnetically attracted to the negative charges on the oxygen atoms of adjacent molecules. This electromagnetic attraction between water molecules, arising from an asymmetrical distribution of the "electron cloud" around the oxygen and hydrogen atoms, is what is termed "hydrogen bonding."

Bridging Waters

The electromagnetic polarity of the water molecule is a property that allows water to participate profoundly in every biochemical activity in the body. Recent research reveals key features of how this property supports water's complex interaction with macromolecules, providing invaluable structural utility. It is known that the structural form of proteins is held together by hydrogen-bonded "water bridges" that link one part of a large molecule to another part. It is the hydrogen bonding property of water, arising from the electromagnetic polarity of the water molecule, that makes this contribution to protein structure possible.

The ubiquitous nature of the watery environment within living things suggests that DNA, RNA, and polysaccharides also are supported in a similar fashion by water. Thus, the structure and function of all biologically active macromolecules depends on the optimal, intimate interaction and integration of water molecules. (Petukhov)

Universal Workhorse

Large bioactive molecular structures, such as proteins, membrane bilayers, chromosomal DNA, and polysaccharides, are always covered with water molecules due to the electromagnetic attraction between water and the hydrophilic (water-loving/attractive) parts of the macromolecules. This intimacy between solute (macromolecules) and solvent (water) draws water into dynamic participation in all biochemical activities. In addition, water acts as a surrounding insulator for macromolecules against electromagnetic interactions from neighboring, electrically charged entities. The polarity of charge on water molecules allows them to adapt readily to local molecular environments.

Protecting Waters

As discussed previously, the cell membrane is composed of a fluid mosaic bilayer of phospholipids, with phosphate groups on the two outside surfaces and fatty acids sandwiched between them. Because of the electromagnetic polarity of the phosphate groups, they attract and hold the polar water molecules (via the positive charge on the hydrogen atoms of water molecules) to both surfaces of the bilayer. Water molecules on the bilayer surfaces, as well as those surrounding them, maintain the structural integrity of the lipid bilayer of cells. They do this by keeping the hydrophilic phosphate groups exposed to the water molecules at the outer surfaces and the hydrophobic (water-avoiding) fatty acid groups sandwiched within the bilayer. Thus, water is absolutely essential to the integrity and functioning of all cell membranes throughout the body.

New Life for an Old Idea

A concept from antiquity is now gaining new respect among modern scientists. According to the ancient Greek philosopher Plato, the basic elements of the universe can be represented by what are now called the "Platonic solids" of geometry: the tetrahedron, cube, octahedron, dodecahedron, and icosahedron. These three-dimensional figures were considered of universal significance, because they were and are the only solid figures structured such that all the corners, centers of the faces, and centers of the edges can touch spheres. Spheres are the three-dimensional symbol of unity and oneness. Plato believed that the element of water was represented by the icosahedron, the 20-sided form that has sides made up of identical, equal-sided triangles. Interestingly, modern researchers are coming to the conclusion that water molecules, under the influence of hydrogen bonding, have a tendency to organize themselves into icosahedron clusters. Plato may have been right after all. (Chaplin)

Many people, including scientists unfamiliar with the structural behavior of water, assume that water is a homogeneous substance in its liquid state. This assumption is absolutely false. According to Martin Chaplin, when in its liquid state, water is a network of relatively large icosahedral clusters.

Chaplin indicates that the size of each icosahedral cluster is three nanometers.

— One nanometer (nm) = one billionth of a meter.

— One angstrom (A) = one ten billionth of a meter.

— Therefore, 1 nm = 10 A.

— Thus, the size of the icosahedral water cluster is 30 angstroms.

If Chaplin and other proponents of the icosahedron model are correct, the major cluster units of liquid water are too large to pass through the aquaporin water channels of the cell membrane, which are only three to six angstroms wide. Therefore, the water channels for the hydration of cells are too small to accommodate the basic cluster structure units of water, allowing water molecules to pass only in a single-file manner.

A question immediately arises: How does water enter the cell if water is clustered in units too large to traverse the cell's aquaporin water channels? By energetic mechanisms not fully understood, the cell membrane and its surrounding layer of water molecules are able to pluck, with blinding speed, individual water molecules from water clusters and move them through the channels.

Clustered Water Gel

To remain in a liquid state rather than gaseous vapor, water molecules must be clustered in groupings with a minimum of five $H2O$ molecules held together by hydrogen bonds. This formation is required, because the vibration frequency of hydrogen will cause a single $H2O$ molecule to become unstable and escape into the gaseous state. The sharing of vibrational energy by several $H2O$ molecules connected by hydrogen bonds allows them to become stable in the form of liquid water.

According to current theory, the smallest structure of liquid water is five H2O molecules hydrogen-bonded in a tetrahedral arrangement. Long-range, weak hydrogen bonds tend to force water molecules to interact with one another, forming large molecular arrays (icosahedral clusters) made up of numerous five H2O-molecule units. These long-range hydrogen bonds constantly are being formed and broken. Hence, water can best be described, especially within the cell, as a "gel" that is in a constant state of transformation. The energetic interaction of water clusters, cell membranes with bonded water molecules, and aquaporins control the hydration of cells.

Caveat Emptor: A Word of Caution

The aquaporin protein water channels are designed to admit only pure water and oxygen. Therefore, to optimally hydrate cells, the only thing that belongs in our drinking water is pure water. Some producers of water products proclaim that the addition of certain chemical additives will render water more easily absorbed by cells. For example, some products are made by adding a "surfactant," which is a soap-like compound that reduces surface tension. Sodium metasilicate and potassium carbonate are two of the most common additives found in surfactant-based water products. The continued ingestion of such products may cause health issues in some people, because the body interprets surfactants as contaminants. Because aquaporins are extremely sensitive to toxins, they will shut down if surfactants are present, actually decreasing cell hydration.

Many good water products are available—just do your homework before selecting one. Inquire as to whether the product is stable in heat and cold and during shipment. Also, look out for undesirable additives. If the product has chemical additives, it is not a pure water product. It is a chemically altered compound, manipulated to lower surface tension. The best way to make sure a product is pure and free of contaminants is to request a complete laboratory analysis from the manufacturer. Any reputable manufacturer will be happy to send you this information. If the manufacturer or bottler does not provide the necessary information from an independent laboratory, try another water company. Web site lab reports, unless unedited, are not credible. When you receive the analysis, pay close attention to levels of chlorine, fluoride, arsenic, mercury, lead, aluminum, and other heavy metal contaminants. Be especially concerned about comments regarding trace amounts of toxins, such as arsenic or mercury. Find out how much is meant by "trace amounts." If it can be measured on a consistent basis within or below report limits, it is not truly a "trace" amount and may cause health problems.

chapter four
Nourishing Water:
Hydrating the Body and Its Cells

Conventional and alternative medical authorities alike emphasize the need to increase water intake to improve health. Many people assume they can substitute other fluids (e.g., coffee, tea, soft drinks, beer, soup, juices) and get the same health benefits. People consume these to quench their thirst and attend to their bodies' need for water. Manufacturers of sports drinks have touted the "wonders" of their products. However, a careful look at the way in which water moves, from the fluids we drink into the bloodstream and our cells, may cause us to rethink our use of these popular beverages as primary hydration sources.

Molecules on the Move

Molecules traverse cells by three means: diffusion, osmosis, and protein-assisted transport. (Berne) We have all observed examples of diffusion in action whenever we detect a spray of perfume dispersing through the air of a room. Perhaps your high school science teacher once illustrated the concept by showing a drop of dark ink plunging and dispersing into a beaker of water. These simple examples demonstrate the movement of molecules in a liquid or gaseous medium from a place where they are in higher concentration to a place where they are in lower concentration. That movement is called "diffusion."

The word osmosis is within the vocabulary of most readers, thanks to science teachers. We often encounter this word in conversation and writing, but few people recall the exact meaning their teachers tried to convey.

To understand osmosis, we must first know something about cell membranes, the entities that separate the watery contents of one cell from another. Some membranes are semipermeable. This means that they control which substances pass through them from the cell's watery exterior to its watery interior. Osmosis is the term for the diffusion of water across a semipermeable membrane. To be more precise, osmosis is the diffusion or passage of water molecules from a region of high water molecule concentration, through a permissive, semipermeable membrane, to a region of low water molecule concentration.

The third way molecules can move across a cell membrane occurs by protein-assisted transport. We already touched on one example of this method when we discussed aquaporins in Chapter Two.

Aquaporins are the protein channels that assist the transport of water molecules across the fatty cell membrane. Aquaporins provide the permeability of cell membranes to water. Therefore, osmosis requires open aquaporins. The aquaporins in some tissues are controlled by activators such as antidiuretic hormone (ADH) and serine (an amino acid) in red blood cells. These activators cause aquaporins, drawn from repositories within the cell, to be installed in the cell membrane as needed. For example, the cell membranes of the kidney collecting ducts are usually impermeable to water, so that excess water is excreted in the urine. However, under the influence of ADH, these cells install aquaporin water channel proteins into their membranes, allowing the return of needed pure water into the cell. Another example occurs when muscle and fat cells are under the influence of insulin. Insulin triggers the installation of glucose transport proteins into these cell membranes to permit the passage of glucose from the blood into the cells.

Given adequate water supplies, the body's hydration systems are very efficient. Far too often, however, we unwittingly thwart the body by ingesting substances that impede hydration.

Things That Get in the Way

To understand the reason some substances may impede hydration, you must be familiar with a concept called "concentration gradient." As stated previously, osmosis is the diffusion or passage of water from a region of high water concentration, through a permissive semipermeable membrane, to a region of low water concentration. The amount of pressure that must be applied against this osmotic movement of water is called "osmotic pressure." This pressure is a measure of how vigorously water is attempting to cross the membrane. It is a direct result of the different levels of water concentration that exist at the various points along the water's path as it moves across the membrane. When charted on a graph, these differences form an incline or decline called a "gradient." Therefore, the term used to describe the differences in water concentration across membranes is "water concentration gradient." The osmotic pressure (i.e., the vigor of water's effort to cross the membrane) is proportional to the concentration gradient. In other words, the higher the water concentration on one side of the membrane relative to the other side, the higher the osmotic pressure.

Any substances dissolved in water outside the cell membrane decrease the concentration of water molecules and, therefore, decrease osmotic pressure. As we have just explained, water movement, vigor, and direction are determined by the strength and direction of the water concentration gradient across the membrane. If the concentration of solutes in the exterior water is less than the concentration of solutes in the interior cell water, the concentration of water molecules is greater outside the cell than inside. Therefore, hydration by osmosis occurs when water molecules move down their concentration gradient from the exterior, where they are more plentiful, to the interior, where they are less plentiful. Conversely, if the concentration of solutes is higher in the exterior than the interior, water molecules are in higher concentration within the cell. For this reason, water molecules will move down their concentration gradient from the interior to the exterior. Thus, the cell becomes dehydrated. (Berne)

Now let's apply these principles to discover the most efficient way to hydrate the body.

Nature's Beverage

The rate at which any beverage can hydrate the body depends on its solute concentration. If the concentration of solutes is low, water can pass easily through the mucous lining of the stomach and small intestine, quickly hydrating the body. Obviously, the beverage with the least amount of solutes and, therefore, the greatest ability to hydrate the body down to the cellular level is pure water.

If anything is dissolved in water (e.g., coffee, tea, sugar, flavorings, colors, protein), the osmotic drive is reduced. Body and cell hydration are, therefore, inhibited by the consumption of beverages

36

containing dissolved substances. Pure water is the beverage of choice for optimal hydration of the body.

Dispelling Myths About Pure Water

It is truly amazing how certain myths and untruths are accepted as facts because of incessant, mind-conditioning repetition and biased opinions devoid of reason or experiential evidence. One such myth is the widely held belief that pure water, without any mineral content, is somehow dangerous to drink. The theory is that pure water will "leach" minerals from the body, depleting nutrient reserves.

In reality, most minerals in the body are stored within tissues and cells as components of biochemical complexes. Pure water cannot simply wash them away. The electrolyte minerals sodium, potassium, and chloride are the least bound to tissue infrastructure and, therefore, subject to rapid depletion via vomiting, diarrhea, and other massive fluid losses. Such losses do not occur from ingesting pure water. Other minerals serve a variety of functions, such as enzyme cofactors, protein structural members, and bone matrix constituents, which require bonded association between minerals and the structures they support. Such integration of minerals into cellular and tissue matrices prevents them from being carried off haphazardly with passing water molecules. This is precisely the reason special chelating agents—compounds that bond with unwanted substances—are needed to dislodge toxic heavy metal ions from the body.

There have been no scientific studies conducted to prove or disprove the concerns about pure water. On the other hand, there is scientific evidence that certain beverage and food choices contribute to mineral deficiency and mineral losses. For example, refined, processed foods cause severe losses of minerals. People derive mineral nutrients from whole, unprocessed foods, such as vegetables, fruits, whole grains, raw nuts and seeds, legumes, and organic animal protein sources. Most Americans do not eat the amounts of these foods required to meet their bodies' needs. In addition, crops grown in soil that is not continuously enriched with natural compost and other nutrient-rich, organic fertilizers are deprived of the full range of mineral nutrients, as are the people who eat them.

People who wish to use unpurified, mineral-containing water as a dietary source of these minerals may be fooling themselves. Many of these water sources have dangerous quantities of toxic substances and fail to provide nutritionally adequate amounts of minerals to be of much benefit. It would take the daily consumption of thousands of cups of water from these sources to even approach the Recommended Daily Allowances (RDAs) of nutrient minerals. Furthermore, even if you were willing to consume such huge quantities of water, the RDAs are not optimal levels for many people. Any arguments in favor of unpurified water as a nutrient source simply "do not hold water."

To make matters worse, soft drinks, commonly consumed as substitutes for pure water, are proving to be a major contributing factor to several diseases. For example, consuming high levels of phosphates found in soft drinks, without counterbalancing calcium levels, lowers serum calcium and increases calcium excretion in the urine. This can contribute to osteoporosis in adults and can increase children's risk for developing impaired calcification of growing bones. There is a significant inverse correlation between serum calcium and the number of bottles of soft drinks consumed per week. Regrettably, the per capita consumption of soft drinks in the United States is at least 150 quarts per year. (Pizzorno)

There is absolutely no substitute for pure, clean water. If our bodies do not receive adequate amounts, we will eventually pay the price.

water

The Foundation of Youth, Health, and Beauty

chapter five
Pure Water: A Threatened Resource

Although at least two-thirds of the Earth is covered with water, only three percent of it is fresh, and only 0.01 percent is accessible to human beings. Annually, three million people succumb to untimely deaths from illnesses linked to contaminated water. Shamefully, at the beginning of the 21st century, two billion members of the human family have virtually no access to clean water.

Vanishing Waters: Dwindling Supply

Humans tend to take for granted whatever is in abundant supply. Water often is taken for granted by many in modern temperate-zone industrialized nations, where turning on the faucet delivers an endless supply. In arid regions, however, adequate water supply and access can mean the difference between agricultural success and failure or between life and death.

In many desert regions of the world, water may soon become as precious as oil. And it is not only in distant lands such as the Sahara or the Middle East that water is in jeopardy. Population pressure in the American Southwest and California have put ever-increasing demands on limited fresh water supplies. In addition, those supplies are contaminated with the waste products of our modern industrial and agricultural civilization. Violent clashes already are occurring between farmers, whose survival depends on using limited river water to irrigate parched patches of land, and fishermen, whose livelihood depends on adequate river water to facilitate the spawning of salmon. (Rothfeder)

Heavy Metals and the Fountain of Youth

Since the dawn of recorded history, human beings have searched for the mythical "Fountain of Youth." The first recorded search for the fabled font of rejuvenation occurred in China during the reign of Emperor Ch'in shih-huang-tif (259 to 210 BC). Having built an empire he hoped would last for ten thousand years, Emperor Ch'in sent his emissaries to the four corners of the world to find the Fountain of Youth, so he might live to enjoy his 10,000-year empire. One of the emissaries returned with a potion said to be the "elixir of youth." Emperor Ch'in consumed the elixir, which was actually mercury, and died shortly thereafter. Thus ended the reign of the most powerful ruler in the known world, and the first recorded death from heavy metal poisoning occurred.

There has always been a universal consciousness that water is the Fountain of Youth, and for good cause. We are water beings; without it, life as we know it cannot exist. In our arrogance, we modern, industrialized humans believe we have surpassed the ignorance of our ancestors, who were so foolish as to drink water laced with heavy metals. Ironically, human beings are being exposed to greater levels of heavy metal toxins today than ever before. The voracious demands of our modern technology have overused ground water, causing the concentration of heavy metals (such as arsenic) to increase in drinking water worldwide.

Gremlins in the Elixir of Life

As with so many other resources, the most dangerous species on the planet relative to the quality and availability of potable water is the human being. The ways in which we adversely affect water resources are numerous, including

— mining release of toxic heavy metals;

— oil and natural gas drilling, accompanied by brine pits;

— residues of underground storage of gasoline and oil;

— agricultural run-off of pesticides and other chemicals;

— deforestation;

— urban drainage systems;

— sewage treatment;

— landfills and other waste disposal;

— septic tanks and cesspools; and

— gasoline and oil storage tanks underground. (A'o)

These common practices have taken their toll on the quality of drinking water. Journalists have been reporting on this problem for decades, but the situation grows worse as ecological stress and water demands increase with the human population.

Clandestine, Insidious Villains

Few of us take the time to ponder what is lurking in our water as we prepare our morning coffee. Yet hidden among the water molecules are a cast of insidious characters with the power to deplete our health. We may not experience their adverse effects in the short term, but over time these poisons accumulate in our tissues, disrupting healthy function and instigating pathological processes.

The following list of toxic contaminants is by no means exhaustive. For a more detailed discussion, see *Don't Drink the Water: The*

Essential Guide to Our Contaminated Drinking Water and What You Can Do About It, by Lono Kahuna Kupua A'o, (Kali Press, 1998).

ARSENIC is a major toxin in many water sources. Arising from natural sources, industrial runoff, and pesticide residues, it is a slow-acting, deadly poison that accumulates in body tissues with the ability to induce malignancy.

CHLORINE is a familiar disinfectant and bleaching agent. Unfortunately, it is also carcinogenic and produces poisonous byproducts. As a substance that can neutralize the efficacy of vitamin E, it has the potential to induce cell damage that accelerates a number of ailments associated with the depletion of the antioxidant protection of vitamin E. These conditions include nerve damage, muscle weakness, and red blood cell fragility. (Murray) In addition, constant exposure of the lower bowel to the antiseptic properties of chlorine may have the same effect as constant exposure to antibiotics—an imbalance in the bacterial microflora in the colon. (A'o)

FLUORIDE is one of the most controversial additives in urban water systems. Although advocated by dentists to retard the development of tooth cavities, the effects on the rest of the body are unfavorable. These include rendering other bone tissue in the body more brittle, inducing carcinogenic influence, and disrupting the function of enzyme systems.

HYDROGEN SULFIDE is an odiferous byproduct of the decay and disintegration of underground organic matter. Although not as poisonous as other toxins, it can be harmful in high doses.

LEAD has been a scourge on human health for ages. Although pipes are no longer made of lead, this heavy metal can still be found in water fixtures and solder materials. As it accumulates in tissues, lead damages the brain, nervous system, and kidneys.

METHYL TERTIARY BUTYLATED ETHER (MTBE) is a gasoline additive that escapes from underground gasoline storage tanks, seeping its way through soil and rock and settling into ground water sources, where it develops an offensive odor and taste. Although its effects on human health have not been thoroughly researched, animal studies suggest that it may be carcinogenic at high doses. The U.S. Environmental Protection Agency (EPA) has yet to set a limit on the amount of MTBE allowed in drinking water.

CHROMIUM (VI) (Cr [VI]) is a byproduct of industrial processes such as forging stainless steel, chrome plating, manufacturing dyes and pigments, tanning leather, producing photographic materials, and staining wood. Particles of Cr (VI) are scattered through the air within and surrounding industrial plants, settling on land and water and eventually sinking into underground aquifers. When Cr (VI) is consumed, body tissues work to convert it to the harmless nutrient Cr (III). A multiplicity of natural barriers also prevent Cr (VI) penetration to deeper organs. This explains why diseases linked to Cr (VI) are confined to tissues at the point of entry. However, continuous Cr (VI) bombardment is undoubtedly a major contributing factor to cancer. Tissue capacity to reduce Cr (VI) to Cr (III) becomes exhausted, leaving tissues susceptible to free radical oxidation, cell damage, and DNA mutations. For this reason, massive Cr (VI) exposure may spawn malignancy.

NITRATES and NITRITES are constituents of farm and suburban fertilizers, as well as livestock waste. These compounds seep into the water table and ride drainage water into rivers, lakes, and streams. Toxic to infants, these compounds are also unhealthy for adults, because natural biochemical processes in the stomach convert these compounds into carcinogenic nitrosamines.

RADON is a radioactive gas that plagues many parts of the United States. Arising from natural underground radioactive mineral deposits, as well as the nuclear decay of uranium mining residues, radon is one of the most dangerous water pollutants, because its radioactive influence can cause many cancer deaths.

NUCLEAR WASTE may become a health nightmare. Deadly radioactive materials with half-lives measured in thousands of years, housed in containers with durability measured in dozens of years, is a recipe for ecological catastrophe of gargantuan proportions. For example, at Hanford, one of the largest nuclear waste dumps in the country, there are already indications that some of the underground containers are beginning to disintegrate. Although massive governmental effort is underway to prevent contamination of the water table and nearby tributaries of the Columbia River, this serves as an example of the potential future threat nuclear waste poses around the world to humanity's most precious natural resources.

Scope of the Problem

In a report issued in July 2001, the EPA revealed that arsenic levels as low as three parts per billion (ppb) increase the risk of skin, bladder, and lung cancer, and may contribute to increased incidence of hypertension, cardiovascular disease, and diabetes. Yet today's standards still remain at 50 ppb—more than 16 times the amount known to cause cancer. Although the government is working to lower the Maximum Level of Contamination (MLC) to the new proposed standard of 10 ppb, this level is still three times the level known to be dangerous.

Government decisions that affect our health are being made, in large part, based on what is affordable for municipalities. Unfortunately, removing arsenic from our drinking water may not fit into the government's financial plan. Interestingly, the EPA's maximum level of contaminates goal (MLCG) is 0.0 ppb. This is a huge problem that will probably not be resolved in our lifetime.

The Natural Resources Defense Council estimates the following odds for increased risk of developing cancer from arsenic in our drinking water.

PPB	Odds
0.5	1 in 10,000
1	1 in 5,000
3	1 in 1,667
4	1 in 1,250
5	1 in 1,000
10	1 in 500
20	1 in 250
25	1 in 200
50	1 in 100

If these were the odds in Lottery games, many of us would be millionaires. Regrettably, this is not the only problem caused by arsenic and heavy metals in drinking water.

Dirty Little Secret

Most people don't realize that the pipes carrying municipal water supplies are themselves sources of contamination. Until recently, the major concrete conduits that carry large quantities of city water were reinforced with asbestos, the toxic fibrous mineral associated with lung and other cancers. Consequently, municipal water supplies carry significant amounts of asbestos fibers. In fact, the contamination is so intense, the EPA has set a quality standard of seven million asbestos fibers per liter.

The leniency of this standard was probably established to accommodate the overwhelming number of asbestos pipes. In fact, hundreds of thousands of miles of conduits throughout the nation would have to be replaced in order to be in accordance with current environmental and occupational safety standards for asbestos, at a cost of many billions of dollars.

Just how toxic asbestos is when ingested rather than inhaled is still being studied; however, the problem needs to be put on the table for public discussion and addressed forthrightly.

Bad Tasting Water

Considering all the pollutants and contaminants listed above, is there any wonder why water often tastes terrible? Sadly, in their efforts to avoid bad-tasting water, many people turn to popular soft drinks. Little do they realize they are simply moving from one source of toxins to another.

The Pause That Does Not Refresh

Soft drink consumption is reaching staggering levels, and much of it is drunk from aluminum cans—a frightening thought when you consider scientists are beginning to recognize a link between aluminum toxicity and Alzheimer's disease.

The acidic constituents of soft drinks and fruit juices enclosed in aluminum cans tend to chemically interact with and erode the aluminum into these beverages. And the results are startling. For example, the canned version of one of the most popular soft drinks in America has been found to contain more than 6,000 ppb of aluminum. This is a staggering amount compared to the EPA maximum of 50 ppb for water. (Municipal water systems run between 40 and 70 ppb.)

Add to this concern the fact that American children have become so accustomed to sweet beverages that more than 70 percent of preschool children drink no water at all. One can only imagine what is happening to their developing tissues if these sweet drinks are served from aluminum cans.

Viable Solutions

What should be done to prevent the problems associated with water pollutants? We now know that the newly discovered aquaporin water channels only permit the influx of pure water and oxygen, so we surmise we can support our cells and prevent disease by consuming abundant quantities of pure water, free of chemicals, heavy metals, sugar, salt, minerals, coffee, teas, soft drinks, and other dissolved substances. Although many of these items may have a place in the diet, they are not what the cell needs and craves for optimal hydration.

To ensure the water you drink is safe, take some measure of personal responsibility. Do not expect the government or industry to provide clean pure water. Do your homework. Investigate what is in your water. Make sure the water you choose is clean and free of heavy metal toxins and undesirable minerals, and that it is biologically safe. Water purity must be a prime concern of all health-conscious people and the government agencies serving their water needs.

water

The Foundation of Youth, Health, and Beauty

chapter six
Rejuvenating Waters:
Hydration for Seniors

Dehydration is one of the most common causes of hospitalization among people over the age of 65, costing the Medicare system an estimated $450 million annually and taking an even greater toll on human life. Half of these people die within one year of admission. Yet there are simple, effective ways to avoid this tragedy, which also can increase vitality, slow the aging process, and make our later years much easier to bear.

Under-hydration in the Elderly

Many factors lead to clinical and subclinical dehydration among seniors, including

— lower body water percentage;

— lack of awareness of hydration needs;

— lack of mental clarity and attentiveness to personal needs;

— illness that accelerates water loss through vomiting, fever, and/or diarrhea; and

— decline of thirst sensation with age.

Water and Aging: The Price of Negligence

When someone looks younger than the average person her age, we tend to say that "the years have been kind." Perhaps it is genetics;

perhaps it has been a life with few cares; or perhaps she has simply been kind to herself in ways the average person has not.

Previous chapters have explained the importance of optimal hydration down to the cellular level, which optimizes metabolic processes throughout the body. In its struggle for survival, the body is designed to alter metabolic processes to compensate for deficits in nutritional intake. If we fail to eat healthy foods and drink adequate amounts of pure water, the body will compensate in order to survive, but a high price is paid. In the absence of sufficient, whole, unprocessed macronutrients (i.e., water, protein, essential fatty acids, complex carbohydrates) and micronutrients (i.e., vitamins, minerals, and cofactors), energy and biochemical resources, which could have been used to maintain youthful tissue integrity and physical vigor, must be redirected. These resources are shifted away from mechanisms that increase longevity toward those that increase the odds for short-term survival. As a result, free-radical damage proliferates, cell and tissue structure is compromised and not as well maintained, metabolic residues and debris accumulate more rapidly within cells, and the process of aging accelerates.

Adequate water supplies within the cell ensure efficient functioning of DNA and mRNA, as well as the maintenance of form and function of structural proteins and enzymes.

Of particular importance in aging are the enzymes that neutralize free radicals. Antioxidant enzyme function demands optimal cell hydration. The water content of cells participates either directly or indirectly in all biochemical reactions. Denying yourself optimal supplies of water accelerates the aging of the body, just as failing to replenish and change oil regularly accelerates the aging of an automobile engine. Negligence leads to unpleasant and untimely long-term consequences.

The Sense That Cannot Be Trusted

As explained previously, the sense of thirst is controlled by thirst cells in the hypothalamus. Thirst occurs after osmoreceptors have sampled the concentration of solutes in the blood and found it to be too high. But the thirst mechanism, even among young, healthy people at the peak of fitness, is not a reliable indicator of the body's water needs. One reason for this dilemma is osmoreceptors are sensitive to certain solutes in the blood (e.g., sodium) and insensitive to others (e.g., urea). A build-up of blood solutes and a decline in blood water content could conceivably go undetected by the osmoreceptors.

Thirst is easily quenched on a temporary basis by a few swallows of fluids acting on moisture receptors in the mouth, throat, and upper gastrointestinal tract. Although thirst will return due to osmoreceptor stimulation, the continuous temporary satiation of thirst with ineffectively small doses of fluids leaves the body in a continuous state of water deficit—a catch-up game the body can never win.

The beverages commonly used to quench thirst (e.g., soft drinks, juices, coffee, tea, beer, cocktails) contain so many dissolved solutes that the movement of water from the gastrointestinal tract into the blood is inhibited and delayed. Optimal hydration is achieved with pure water. As we age, the already unreliable sense of thirst becomes even less sensitive. Senior citizens cannot trust their sense of thirst to tell them when their bodies need water.

Experimental Evidence

The effect of dehydration on the aging sense of thirst was tested in a study comparing the responses of elderly men, age 67 to 75 years, and young men, 20 to 31 years. After a period of water deprivation, the older men had greater increases in plasma solutes, sodium concentration, and ADH levels than the younger men. Yet, the older men were less thirsty and drank less after water deprivation than the younger men. The older men did not drink enough to dilute their plasma and urine to the levels that existed before dehydration. Researchers concluded that after water deprivation, "there is a deficit in thirst and water intake in healthy elderly men, as compared with younger men." (Phillips) This is true despite the fact that ADH response is maintained.

These challenging realities mandate vigilance on the part of senior citizens and the people who assist them in ensuring adequate hydration throughout the day. As indicated previously, the daily intake of pure water should be the number of fluid ounces equal to one-half the number of pounds of body weight. The total amount calculated should be distributed throughout the day and consumed in small doses every 15 or 20 minutes to ensure continuous, optimal hydration. This kind of intake helps prevent health crises involving fainting and collapse due to dehydration commonly seen among the elderly.

Perils From the Faucet

Civil servants who purify water for public use via municipal water systems do the best job they can with the resources they have. Nevertheless, a recent study conducted and published by researchers in the Environmental Epidemiology Program at the Harvard School of Public Health indicates the adverse effects of city drinking water on senior citizens. (Schwartz) The researchers found a close correlation between cloudy (turbid) tap water and hospital admissions of seniors with gastrointestinal complaints in a major American city.

Researchers concluded the elderly residents of that city are at risk for waterborne, gastrointestinal diseases because of current water treatment practices. Moreover, in their opinion, those seeking hospital care represent a very small percentage of the total number of people adversely affected by these circumstances. Because the immune function, disease resistance, and recuperative powers of senior citizens are weaker than in younger individuals, the elderly are extremely sensitive to less than ideal drinking water quality. For this reason, seniors and their caregivers must insist on the purest water available.

chapter seven
Laughing Waters: Hydration for Athletes

Water and Athletic Performance

Now that we have a grasp on the many ways water assists the body and its cells, let's apply what we have learned to the hydration needs of the athlete.

Optimal hydration is paramount to maximum performance because of the following functions performed by water.

— Stabilization of body temperature

— Removal of lactic acid and waste products from muscle cells

— Maintenance of DNA/mRNA structure and function for the generation of new repair proteins

— Support of the three-dimensional infrastructure of enzymes that repair existing proteins

— Reinforcement of protein structure

— Facilitation of the reactions in the cell mitochondria that release energy from the energy currency molecule, known as ATP

— Transport of compounds made in the central nervous system to the periphery

— Transport of nutrients and oxygen to cells throughout the body

In addition, water serves as the major constituent in the synovial fluid in joints; the fluids between the lungs and the chest wall and the abdominal organs and the inner lining of the abdomen; the cushioning material in cartilage and vertebral disks that absorbs the shock of forces generated during vigorous movement; and the connective tissue fluids that lubricate movements of muscles and fascia.

To Err Is Human, Even Among Olympians

One of the strange characteristics of athletes, even elite, world-class performers, is the tendency to underestimate the amount of water their bodies lose during workouts and competitions. Hydration is particularly problematic for athletes, because they perspire more freely than nonathletes. This issue has received special attention at recent national conferences and symposia on athletic performance. The loss of one and one half quarts of water, a common amount for athletes to lose during performance, results in a 25 percent loss of stamina.

It seems ironic that individuals totally attuned to their bodies and focused on maximum physical output so frequently misjudge the amount of water required to replace the water lost in training and tournament. By drinking too little, too infrequently, many athletes not only deny themselves and their fans their peak performance, they unnecessarily threaten their health and well-being.

As discussed previously, the underlying problem may be that the sense of thirst is easily satiated by amounts of water too small to hydrate the body. Temporary satiation occurs before water even enters the bloodstream. However, thirst soon returns, because the osmoreceptors in the hypothalamus are still detecting high concentrations of solutes in the blood. Unfortunately, if an athlete continues to perform until thirst returns, he or she can lose substantial amounts of water via sweat, while taking in small, inadequate amounts of water to satiate the fickle and unreliable sense of thirst. This inadvertent, self-imposed dehydration is one of the main reasons it can take so long for athletes to recover from intense workouts and competitions. Adequate hydration reduces recovery time and enhances performance.

Even among Olympic champions, the sense of thirst cannot be trusted to measure hydration, especially at the cellular level. The hydration of an athlete's body must be as disciplined and structured within the order of training regimens as any other aspect of athletic practice and performance.

What Every Athlete Must Know

None of the benefits of optimal hydration can be enjoyed by an athlete unless water molecules move efficiently from the gastrointestinal tract to the bloodstream, and from the bloodstream to the interior of the cells. As discussed in previous chapters, water moves through tissues in accordance with the physiologic principles of diffusion and osmosis, as well as the structural anatomy and biochemical properties of cell membranes. The following are the most salient points to remember.

— Water molecules diffuse (travel) down their concentration gradient from a region of high water molecule concentration to a region of low water molecule concentration.
— Osmosis is the diffusion of water molecules through a permissive, semipermeable membrane.
— The concentration of water molecules in solution (mixed with dissolved substances) is less than the concentration of water molecules in pure water.

For this reason, whenever solutes are dissolved in water, the osmotic force that drives water molecules to diffuse through semipermeable membranes is reduced. Thus, solutes inhibit the efficiency of osmosis.

A Rational Approach to Athletic Hydration

Physical exertion places high metabolic demands on the body that need to be addressed with the help of a judicious nutritional regimen. When making intelligent choices that best serve the needs of the body under athletic stress, consider the unique metabolism of the individual athlete, the type of physical activity involved, the duration of the activity, and the atmospheric temperature and other conditions under which the activity takes place.

Athletically fit people naturally perspire more freely on average than those living sedentary lives. Water losses in perspiration and urine are necessary to meet certain physiological needs. For example, perspiration is part of the body's cooling system. Dehydration associated with exercise increases core body temperature, heart and respiratory rates, and body fluid concentration of solutes. It also decreases body fluid volumes. (Kelly) The fluid loss that occurs through perspiration is controlled by metabolism, atmospheric temperature, and humidity. And, of course, for optimal performance, the athlete must begin the activity in a state of full hydration. Hydration should continue throughout the activity to satisfy optimal cell water needs and control elevations in core body temperature. When choosing rehydration products, consider the amount of water, electrolytes, and carbohydrates your body needs.

Effect of Exercise on Water in the Athlete's Body

For the average person engaging in moderate physical activity, rehydration is the major consideration. Pure water in adequate quantities is quite sufficient to maintain biochemical balance before, during, and after exertion. The kinds of activities for which water is sufficient include, but are not limited to, moderate-intensity walking, biking, running, swimming, and weight training. Exercise in conditions of high atmospheric temperature increases the potential for dehydration and requires extra vigilance to maintain adequate water intake. (Terrados)

High-intensity exercise, such as the kind performed by endurance athletes, requires a balanced intake of water and carbohydrate-electrolyte replacement to minimize adverse physiological disturbances induced by severe physical exertion. Studies indicate that for high-intensity workouts lasting up to three hours in the heat, both water and carbohydrate-electrolyte drinks provide equivalent benefits in terms of rectal temperature, heart rate, and sweat rate during exercise. However, carbohydrate-electrolyte sources may provide more benefit during immediate recovery because of their ability to quickly replenish glycogen stores. (Carter, Maughan) Carbohydrate consumption alone within one hour after exercise also can restore muscle glycogen rapidly. Although quantities must be adequate to the task, the form (liquid or solid) and presence of other macronutrients does not affect the rate of glycogen restoration. (Kelly, Burke)

Hydration Efficiency

The efficacy of a given drink is limited by the rate of absorption of fluid from the intestines, which is in turn limited by gastric emptying. (Kelly) The issue of absorption efficiency lies at the heart of the question concerning the kind of beverage that best suits a specific purpose. If the desired end is simply water replacement, then nothing will hydrate more efficiently than pure water. However, for carbohydrate-electrolyte drinks, gastric emptying is an issue, because the digestive process is involved. Several factors influence gastric emptying, including exercise intensity; the concentration of carbohydrates and salts in the solution; the caloric content, volume, temperature, and pH of the ingested fluid; the metabolic state and biochemical individuality of the athlete; and the temperature of the environment. (Neufer, Rehrer)

The Dangers of Sugary Sports Drinks

The marketplace is replete with competitive, glitzy advertising for sugary sports drinks, but a word of caution is needed here. These beverages are sugar-based drinks that rapidly increase blood sugar. Such an increase gives rise to an outpouring of insulin from the pancreas, as well as increased levels of chromium, niacin, and other nutrients to ensure adequate insulin receptor response by muscle and fat cells. In order to avoid problems caused by persistently high insulin levels, such as the deposit of glucose into fat cells, it is wise to limit consumption of these products to the first hour of postexercise recovery. It also is strongly recommended that you combine them with pure water if consumed during events lasting more than two or three hours. A sugary beverage consumed immediately before exercise may actually impair performance. The large insulin response induced by a rapid increase in blood sugar may cause hypoglycemia (i.e., low blood sugar) during exercise. (Kelly) Use pure water immediately before an event to maximize hydration.

Optimizing Long-Term Recovery

After muscle glycogen stores have been replenished, other muscle tissue needs also should be addressed within the first hour after exercise to minimize exercise stress. One of the most important of these is the exercise-induced, microtrauma tears to muscle fibers. The rapid generation of repair protein depends on optimal hydration of DNA, mRNA, protein-manufacturing structures (e.g., endoplasmic reticulum), and repair enzymes. Quick repair of microtrauma demands ideal muscle cell hydration. Another important factor is the accumulation of lactic acid in muscle tissue. Lactic acid is a metabolic byproduct produced when muscle tissue is pushed into anaerobic levels of exertion. Inefficient removal of lactic acid can be a source of muscle soreness and fatigue that limits long-term athletic excellence.

To flush lactic acid out of muscle cells efficiently, those cells must be optimally hydrated. Only pure water has the ability to enter the cells in molecular numbers great enough to meet this challenge. Additionally, exercise generates free radicals, which can damage tissues and accelerate the aging process. In addition to dietary antioxidant enzymes, cells have intrinsic antioxidant enzymes that neutralize free radicals as they are generated. However, cellular dehydration impairs enzyme function. Thus, rapid rehydration at the cellular level after exercise is imperative to minimize free radical damage. It is clear that for a host of reasons, athletes should thoroughly and continuously rehydrate with pure water to accelerate post-workout recovery. Some experts recommend weighing yourself before and after a workout. For every pound of weight lost, drink two eight-ounce cups of water to ensure adequate rehydration. (Bird)

chapter eight
Nurturing Waters:
Hidden Hazards of Winter Dehydration

Many people who are careful about drinking enough water during the hot summer months tend to be less vigilant during the winter. Whether you are an athlete or an armchair quarterback, your need to attend to hydration after the temperatures fall is every bit as important as it is during the summer. Winter dehydration can be an insidious contributor to health problems associated with cold weather. Children and the elderly are at the greatest risk.

Naturally, proper winter hydration must not be considered a substitute for using good judgment and common sense when choosing appropriate clothing. Layering and covering the head and extremities to minimize heat loss, as well as sturdy, water-resistant footgear and outer layers are always recommended during inclement weather.

Winter Water Losses

The human body loses water in many ways during winter. For example, although it may not seem as pronounced, exercising in cold weather still causes the body to lose substantial amounts of water through sweating. Cold, winter air cannot hold as much moisture as warm air; therefore, drier air draws more water from the lungs as we breathe. In addition, interior environments are usually very dry in the winter due to drying heating methods. The decreased interior humidity also increases water loss from the lungs and skin.

When the body becomes chilled, blood is shifted away from the periphery (i.e., arms, legs, skin) toward the interior organs to preserve vital heat for these life-sustaining tissues. The directing of blood to the interior increases its flow to the kidneys, automatically increasing the kidney filtration rate and urine output. This effect is called "cold diuresis." Cold weather increases body metabolism and associated water needs required to maintain healthy body temperature.

Respiratory illnesses associated with winter, such as the common cold and influenza, cause the body to generate large amounts of mucous in an effort to rid itself of the offending microbes. The water in these discharges must be replaced. Intestinal influenza, leading to diarrhea and vomiting, requires additional water and, perhaps, electrolyte replacement. We recommend four to eight additional cups daily.

Dehydration and Hypothermia

Dehydration and hypothermia form a potentially lethal combination. Each worsens the other, accelerating the downward spiral toward a serious crisis. Dehydration contributes to hypothermia, because proper hydration helps to optimize blood flow, which circulates heat throughout the body. In addition, the body's water supply has a relatively stable temperature, which helps the body maintain appropriate levels of heat. If a person is dehydrated, this temperature modulating mechanism is not available. Hypothermia worsens dehydration by increasing the loss of water via urine output (i.e., cold diuresis).

Winter Skin Worries

The skin is the largest organ in the human body and the first to feel the effects of cold and dehydration. As previously discussed, exposure to cold temperatures causes the body to direct blood away from the skin toward the inner organs. Dehydration worsens this problem. Blood vessels supplying the skin are constricted to conserve heat and water evaporation. Perspiration and sebum (i.e., skin oil) secretion are reduced, causing the skin to become dry and wrinkled. The production of cellular repair protein, which maintains healthy skin tissue and depends on adequate cell hydration, is reduced in proportion to the skin cell's state of dehydration. Topical moisturizing creams only address the symptoms of dehydration. The problem can only be solved by ingesting the proper cell nutrients—namely, pure water, essential fatty acids, and moderate amounts of vitamins A, C, E, and zinc.

Winter Water Intake

As previously mentioned, the number of fluid ounces of pure water that an average person should drink in a day should equal half of one's body weight in pounds. Thus, a 150-pound person should drink 75 fluid ounces (about 10 eight-ounce glasses) of pure water throughout the day. One should drink more based on physical exertion and losses from perspiration. Many people will be pleasantly surprised to find that pure water is one of their dearest friends as they endeavor to survive the harsh winter elements.

chapter nine
Healing Waters: The "Water Cure"

The Most Overlooked and Underrated Remedy of All

You could ask scores of healthcare professionals about the healing powers of water, and not one in a thousand would be able to discuss them intelligently. Water seems too simple, primitive, and mundane to be worthy of serious consideration by those well-schooled in the mechanistic precision of modern, high-tech medicine. How could water, the blandest substance on earth, be of any value in healing that which ails human beings?

Although not as skeptical as most, the authors of this book had to surrender some preconceived notions about the real value of water in health and healing to fully grasp water's therapeutic potential. Even the author who is a naturopathic physician, thoroughly grounded in concepts of scientifically verified, natural interventions for healing and optimizing wellness, had to be educated in the latest science concerning water's essential chemical characteristics and cell hydration principles, as well as the role of optimal cell hydration in maintaining robust health.

Costly Oversight

Dehydration is a deficiency of optimal water levels within the body and its cells. Dehydration, clinical or subclinical, results from inadequate water intake compared to water loss. As fluids outside cells lose their water content, the concentration of water in these extracellular fluids declines. By osmosis, water molecules move down their concentration gradient from the place where they are more abundant (within the cells), to the place where they are less abundant (the dehydrated extracellular fluids), in order to re-establish osmotic balance. Regrettably, the loss of water from the interior of the cells produces a state of dehydration that impairs all cell functions. Intracellular dehydration can impair the entire process of life by disrupting structural integrity and functional efficacy of all cell components throughout the body.

Cell dehydration obstructs accurate transcription of DNA code sequences to mRNA. Cell dehydration also prevents efficient production of amino acid sequences for protein assembly into cell structural and functional components, such as microtubules and microfilaments, membrane protein channels, membrane receptors for hormones, and other bioactive compounds, such as enzymes that catalyze all biochemical reactions in the body. In addition, toxins accumulate in the body due to a lack of sufficient water for adequate elimination of waste materials.

Now consider a few of the long-term consequences of continuous cell dehydration:
— cell structural disintegration;
— impaired flow of nutrients into the cell due to compromised membrane protein channels;
— local tissue resistance to endocrine hormones due to faulty integrity and responsiveness of membrane receptors;
— chronic fatigue due to lack of enzyme-catalyzed energy production;
— free radical damage of cell structures, including DNA, due to

reduced free radical scavenging;

— inadequate repair of nuclear DNA damage due to faulty enzyme repair activity; and

— reduced production of key bioactive compounds, such as hormones, digestive enzymes, and neurotransmitters.

Multiple Organ System Effects of Dehydration

The stress of dehydration forces the body into a mode of desperate reactivity for survival, which affects a number of organ systems. The survival mode in the central nervous system can be triggered by either emotional stress or the stress of dehydration. In its efforts to maintain water content of approximately 85 percent within brain cells (neurons), the central nervous system reacts to water deficit as a threat to the body's survival. The production of histamine within the central nervous system is increased. (Kjaer) As a result, ADH is released from the pituitary gland to reabsorb water from urine in the collecting ducts of the kidney.

In addition, corticotropin-releasing hormone (CRH) from the hypothalamus triggers the release of adreno-corticotropin (ACTH) from the pituitary. Adreno-corticotropin stimulates the secretion of the hormone cortisol by the adrenal glands. Long-term elevated cortisol

— decreases bone formation and increases bone breakdown,

— decreases muscle mass,

— increases water filtration into the urine,

— decreases connective tissue,

— increases blood pressure,

— inhibits inflammatory responses, and

— inhibits immune response. (Berne)

Adverse Outcomes

Many will find it hard to swallow that long-term subclinical dehydration can contribute to accelerated aging and life-threatening illnesses. However, the numerous consequences of neglecting adequate hydration can interact in a multiplicative way to cause tragic results. For example, uncontrolled free radical damage, inadequate DNA repair, and weakened immune response can combine into a complex that may contribute to the development of cancer. Faulty membrane receptor construction can contribute to such tissue resistant hormonal disorders as Type II adult onset diabetes mellitus. Errors in receptor synthesis also can lead the immune system to mistake cell membrane proteins for foreign invaders, triggering autoimmune attacks on the body's own tissues. This problem is compounded by the inappropriate union of glucose (i.e., blood sugar) molecules with cell membrane proteins, due to high intake of refined carbohydrates (sugar and white flour).

Enter the "Water Doctor"

It has been said that even under the worst conditions, the wise can always find a means to do good. This saying applies very well to an Iranian medical doctor named Fereydoon Batmanghelidj, MD. Born into a prominent family in Tehran, he was educated in the United Kingdom. After returning to his native land, his professional career involved the establishment of medical facilities for the disadvantaged. When the revolutionary government came to power in 1979, Dr. Batmanghelidj was imprisoned, charged with crimes against the new government, and sentenced to death. In a miraculous turn of events, the prison officials found his medical skills useful for attending to the needs of the other prisoners and delayed his execution.

Deprived of his customary medicines, Dr. Batmanghelidj was forced to use the materials at hand. He subsequently discovered the astounding power of a healing tool that was readily available— water. For the next 25 months, he conducted research on the medical uses of water behind the prison walls. When a judge was presented with Batmanghelidj's report on his medical discoveries, the doctor's death sentence was rescinded. He subsequently escaped from Iran and found asylum in the West. Dr. Batmanghelidj has worked ever since on expanding awareness about water's healing powers among fellow professionals and the public. He has written two books on the subject: *Your Body's Many Cries for Water* (Global Health Solutions, 1995) and *ABCs of Asthma, Allergies and Lupus* (Global Health Solutions, 1995).

The "Water Cure"

We wish to be absolutely clear about the power of water: It cures nothing except dehydration. However, once dehydration has been corrected at the cellular level, healing is possible. As indicated in the disclaimer at the beginning of this book, we recommend that any medical interventions contemplated by a patient be undertaken with the full supervision and counsel of a qualified healthcare professional. Before examining water's specific effects on certain ailments, it is necessary to review concepts discussed in previous chapters.

Humans are basically water beings, occupying a planet covered mostly with water, but residing in the planet's most arid environment. Because water is so much a part of who we are as physical beings, our bodies require optimal, continual replenishment of water, which escapes through daily metabolic processes. Our bodies exert tremendous amounts of energy to maintain adequate hydration.

Any deviation from an ideal state of hydration can have profoundly adverse effects all over the body. Less than adequate hydration forces the entire body, and every cell therein, into exhaustive and wasteful modes of compensating behavior in order to survive.

This effort to compensate for less than optimal hydration wastes vital energy and biochemical resources. It is an unnecessary expenditure of precious reserves that accelerates the aging process and decreases longevity. It also leaves us more susceptible to diseases that may be part of our genetic inheritance but are preventable or controllable through conscientious attention to the nutritional needs of each cell in our bodies.

Optimizing hydration at the cellular level helps improve DNA function, mRNA transcription of the DNA code, and protein synthesis and function. In addition, adequate hydration improves the delivery of nutrients and oxygen to the cells and the elimination of carbon dioxide, toxins, and metabolic waste products from the cells and the entire organism. These beneficial effects can only enhance the body's innate ability to heal itself. In naturopathic medicine, we call this "the Healing Power of Nature." With the gradual age-related decline in thirst sensitivity, we tend to become less aware of the body's continuing need for water replenishment. It could be argued that in our failure to attend to the most basic nutritional survival need, we become unwitting participants in our own undoing. We contribute to our own untimely demise by failing to attend to the most elementary requirements of the human body.

Dehydration and Chronic Illness: A Hidden Cause of Suffering

Dr. Batmanghelidj's revolutionary discoveries shed new light on a crucial underlying contributor to many chronic ailments. According to his research, the suffering associated with many disorders is triggered or worsened by dehydration. The reason for this effect is that, under the stress of dehydration, the body takes desperate measures to conserve water. Part of dehydration management involves the release of histamine. (Kjaer) It appears that histamine release is critical to activating other systems designed to save body water.

All of these systems are involved in keeping water in the body at all costs and distributing it to the most critical organs to ensure survival. But there is a price to be paid for these extreme measures. Many of the compounds in the water-conservation systems can worsen symptoms associated with chronic diseases, such as asthma, allergies, and the chronic pain of many long-term disorders. Unfortunately, most healthcare professionals and patients have not recognized the suffering that accompanies these ailments as an indicator of dehydration. Instead, they have turned to pharmaceutical interventions that suppress the symptoms and produce undesirable side effects, rather than treating the hidden factor of dehydration. Until dehydration is corrected, the underlying problem and its pathological consequences remain.

As we stated at the beginning of this chapter, water cures nothing except dehydration. However, when dehydration has been resolved at the cellular level, where the disease process is played out, the healing process can begin naturally. This explains why the results of treating chronic ailments with water have seemed almost miraculous. Restoring cells to optimal pure water content finally addresses the body's desperate biochemical need for water. This intervention allows many health crises to resolve naturally.

Water's Essential Healing Principles

Dr. Batmanghelidj has said, "Chronic cellular dehydration painfully and prematurely kills. Its initial outward manifestations have until now been labeled as diseases of unknown origin." According to Dr. Batmanghelidj, recurrent, noninfectious conditions associated with pain and discomfort in various parts of the body, which cannot be explained by other identifiable causes, should be interpreted as expressions of water deficits at the site of the tissue and cells manifesting the symptoms. In other words, if the cause of suffering cannot be identified, one should consider the possibility that the part of the body showing symptoms is dehydrated. He calls this phenomenon "local thirst." Until local water needs are met, suffering continues.

The range of chronic illnesses Dr. Batmanghelidj has treated with water include

— coronary heart disease,
— peptic ulcers,
— arthritis,
— hypertension,
— low-back pain,
— intermittent claudication (i.e., leg pain due to poor circulation),
— migraine headache,
— hangover headache,
— colitis (i.e., colon inflammation),
— constipation,
— obesity,
— edema (i.e., swelling) of unknown origin or linked to allergies,
— fibromyalgia, and
— chronic fatigue syndrome.

The main precaution to take when using water as a healing intervention is to ensure a patient's kidneys are functioning adequately to allow the passive exit of water from the body as urine. If the kidney filtration units (i.e., glomeruli) are damaged or dysfunctional, the excretion of water via urine is impaired, causing water to be retained in the bloodstream, leading to increased blood pressure.

water

The Foundation of Youth, Health, and Beauty

chapter ten
Healing Waters: Specific Applications

Coronary Heart Disease and Heart Attack

It has been known for some time that high blood and plasma viscosity (thickness), high hematocrit (i.e., percentage of blood that is occupied by cells), and high levels of fibrinogen (i.e., precursor to the fibrous mesh of blood clots) are well correlated with coronary heart disease. Remarkably, even "high-normal" levels of these parameters are considered independent risk factors. Some researchers consider these factors as harmful as smoking, high blood pressure, and high LDL cholesterol. Viscosity, hematocrit, and fibrinogen are often found to be elevated years before the appearance of major circulatory events. They are also implicated in the early stages and development of atherosclerosis, as well as the prognosis of patients diagnosed with atherosclerosis. These factors also have been linked to intermittent claudication. High hematocrit has been associated with tachycardia (i.e., rapid heartbeat), magnitude of heart tissue damage from heart attack, reduced oxygen transport, and reduced blood supply to heart tissue. (Chan)

Only recently have health conditions related to blood thickness been examined in relation to subclinical dehydration. It is unfortunate that the term "blood thinners" has been applied to pharmaceutical anticoagulants, because they are not really thinning agents. Instead, they affect the biochemical processes that allow blood to clot. If paint is too thick, we add paint thinner. If soups, sauces, or gravies are too thick, we add water. In each case, we add more solvent. Blood is a water-based fluid; therefore, to really thin the blood, we need to add pure water. The power of this simple wisdom has only recently been revealed.

Researchers recently analyzed six years' worth of data to determine what influence the consumption of water and other beverages has on the risk of fatal heart attack. The database includes lifestyle choices of more than 8,000 men and 12,000 women aged 25 and older, and notes what factors seemed to correlate with the 246 fatal heart attacks that occurred in this group during that period. The results are striking.

Men who drink five or more glasses of water daily are only 46 percent as likely to have a heart attack as those who drink only two glasses per day. Women who drink five or more glasses are 59 percent as likely to suffer such heart problems. Even more remarkable, compared to those who drink two or fewer glasses of nonwater fluids per day, women who drink five or more have a 147 percent greater risk of heart attack, and men have a 46 percent greater risk. Moreover, these relative risk relationships hold true regardless of adjustments for any other factors.

According to researchers, including cardiologists and public health experts, failing to drink enough water can be as harmful to heart health as smoking. Just by increasing pure water intake, one can reduce risk of death from heart attack by half. This amount of benefit may be greater than that gained by smoking cessation, reducing cholesterol, exercising, or maintaining ideal body weight. According to one researcher, increasing intake of pure water could be the cheapest and simplest method of reducing fatal heart attack risk. (Chan)

Peptic Ulcers and Dyspepsia

The first conditions that brought hidden, subclinical dehydration to the attention of Dr. Batmanghelidj were peptic ulcers and dyspepsia. He has treated thousands of such cases with water therapy. Anecdotal substantiation of the efficacy of this approach is mounting. Chronic inflammation of the stomach and duodenum with associated heartburn and acid reflux are prime indications for water intervention. The concept here is not far-fetched when we understand how digestive organs function.

As discussed earlier, the gastrointestinal tract produces a large quantity of water-based secretions. In addition to producing fluids that carry enzymes for food digestion, the lining (i.e., mucous membrane) of these organs must protect itself from being damaged and digested by its own secretions and those of the pancreas. Mucous produced by the membrane is designed to provide needed protection. However, this water-based, protective material cannot be secreted in sufficient quantities when a person is in a state of subclinical dehydration. This deficit leaves the mucous lining exposed to stomach acid and digestive enzymes that cause inflammation, ulcers, and bleeding. In addition, water deficits reduce the volume of bicarbonate-containing fluids released from the pancreas, which neutralize stomach acid in the duodenum. Water shortage also inhibits the efficient digestion of food, because the digestive enzymes of the small intestine are carried in a water-based medium.

According to Dr. Batmanghelidj, dyspepsia (i.e., digestive upset) is the thirst signal of the gastrointestinal tract. He also has successfully applied water therapy to alleviate the symptoms of colitis and hiatal hernia. Additional anecdotal support is arising from other sources.

Osteoarthritis

Osteoarthritis involves the erosion of cartilage tissue in the weight-bearing joints (e.g., hips, knees), which progresses at a rate faster than the cartilage can be replaced.

Inside the joints are synovial membranes, which produce synovial fluid in sufficient quantity to lubricate the movement of cartilage attached to bone. In a state of subclinical dehydration, the distribution of water may shift away from the joints to tissues more vital to survival. Thus, water shortage can cause insufficient production of synovial fluid and contribute to osteoarthritis.

In addition, the biochemical constituents of joint cartilage (e.g., chondroitin sulfate) are designed to attract and hold water molecules. Water provides the cushioning needed to handle the shock of daily weight-bearing movements. Because cartilage tissue lacks a direct blood supply, water molecules must diffuse through many surrounding structures if they are to distribute themselves effectively. Subclinical dehydration can deprive cartilage tissue of water. Pure water is the most efficient way to hydrate cartilage tissue.

Healthcare professionals and patients would be wise to add pure water to their regimen of glucosamine sulfate and other nutritional remedies for osteoarthritis.

Hypertension

As the body's state of hydration declines, blood volume decreases. This reduction in blood volume then causes a decrease in blood pressure. In an effort to maintain the blood pressure necessary to supply the brain and peripheral tissues, the kidneys release renin into the bloodstream. Renin triggers the generation of the compound angiotensin II, which

— constricts arterioles,

— induces the kidneys (via the adrenal hormone, aldosterone) to retain salt and accompanying water from the urine, and

— stimulates water absorption from the urine in the collecting ducts by inducing the release of ADH. (Berne)

The combined effect of all these actions, which are initiated by inadequate hydration, is a dramatic increase in blood pressure.

Pharmaceutical interventions often are focused on inhibiting the enzyme that produces angiotensin II. However, if the underlying problem is really dehydration, Dr. Batmanghelidj's approach of increasing pure water intake to levels that maintain favorable blood volume is a simpler, safer, and more cost-effective option. Surely this approach should be tried before resorting to more drastic means.

Low Back Pain

The skeletal structure of the human spinal column is a wondrous feat of biological architecture. However, the optimal functioning of this dynamic edifice depends on the functional integrity of the structures that allow movement between the bony vertebrae, while supporting their share of body weight. These structures are the intervertebral disks, which are made up of the nucleus pulposus, or the mucous-like core of the disk; and the anulus fibrosus or the fibrous connective tissue ring that holds the nucleus in place.

In a fashion similar to cartilage, the biochemical constituents of the nucleus pulposus are such that they attract and hold water. This property is essential, because each nucleus pulposus and the water it contains comprise a major weight-bearing unit of the vertebral column. The vertical weight-bearing position of the spine during daily activities squeezes water out of the nucleus pulposus, which must be replaced during sleep while the body is in a nonweight-bearing, horizontal position.

In the absence of adequate hydration, the body cannot replenish water in the vertebral column. Thus, the nucleus and entire disk are flattened by the weight of the body above the disk, pressing the bony vertebrae downward against the nerve roots that exit both sides of the spinal cord.

This problem most severely affects the disk carrying the most weight—the fifth lumbar disk at the bottom of the spinal column—and is a likely source of low back pain. Corrective measures include increased water intake, as well as interventions by a skilled professional (e.g., naturopath, chiropractor, osteopath) experienced in providing the appropriate traction techniques to draw water back into the nucleus pulposus.

Asthma and Allergies

Histamine is a prime mediator of allergy and asthma. It is generated in the central nervous system when the body is dehydrated. It also is released by mast cells located on the mucous membranes of the respiratory and gastrointestinal systems. Histamine works with the immune system, facilitating the movement of white blood cells to sites of microbe invasion. Animal studies indicate that increasing water consumption decreases histamine. As a result, asthma and allergy symptoms are reduced.

Dr. Batmanghelidj has seen this benefit of water demonstrated in scores of patients. Anecdotal evidence from practitioners and patients across the nation is confirming his findings. Of course, identifying and eliminating allergens is the first step in any allergy intervention, followed by the addition of vitamin B12, omega-3 fatty acids, flavonoids, and botanical medicines. Pure water also should be a key component of regimens for states of hypersensitivity, such as asthma and allergy.

Of particular note is the case of exercise-induced asthma. Recent studies indicate that dehydration during exercise can increase the intensity of asthma symptoms in people subject to asthmatic attacks. Dehydration increases the occurrence of spasms in bronchial smooth muscle due to overly dry airway membranes. Dehydration of mucous membranes occurs before an asthmatic athlete even begins training. Dehydrated asthmatics begin exercise with reduced hydration capacity; therefore, a pathological respiratory state occurs more rapidly.

Researchers have concluded that, "Exercise-induced asthma is an exaggerated airway response to airway dehydration." (Medrala) Airway narrowing from exercise in elite athletes and otherwise healthy subjects now is considered a physiologic response to pathologic changes in airway cells resulting from "dehydration injury." These changes occur in healthy subjects exercising intensely for long periods, breathing cold air, dry air, or both. (Anderson)

To minimize risk of asthmatic attack during exercise, it is imperative for athletes to be in a state of optimal hydration and to maintain good hydration status throughout the exercise and during recovery. Pure water can be a very dear friend to an asthmatic.

Edema: Silent Destroyer

Edema describes swelling that occurs when excess fluids accumulate in the connective tissue between capillaries and cells. Edema is a symptom of underlying health issues and not a disease category unto itself. Depending on the cause, edema may be confined to localized tissues or may affect the entire body. (Collins)

The following factors and disease states can give rise to edema.
— Capillary injury
— Hypersensitivity reactions
— Heart failure
— Kidney failure
— Vascular abnormalities
— Allergies
— Adverse reactions to medicines
— Exercise
— Premenstrual syndrome
— Pregnancy
— High altitude
— Low blood proteins
— Adrenal disorders
— Liver cirrhosis
— Tumors

Prompt examination by a qualified healthcare professional is imperative to determine the underlying cause of edema. Self-diagnosis can be very dangerous. However, if edema is part of a professionally diagnosed, hypersensitivity condition, hydration may be a helpful component of an effective intervention protocol. Edema often is associated with food allergies and other hypersensitivity reactions.

Therefore, in addition to allergen identification and avoidance as well as other interventions, optimizing hydration may be one of the simplest and most effective treatments available.

Mainstream medical approaches to edema employ diuretics and a reduction in fluid intake, which can be extremely counter-productive in many cases. Diuretics reduce edema but do not address the underlying causes. Reducing fluid intake is not only counter-productive, it also is dangerous to the overall health of the body.

In addition to issues associated with hypersensitivity, subclinical dehydration permits the accumulation of discarded toxins and debris in the connective tissues. When this happens, there is a high concentration of waste products and a low concentration of water molecules. When fresh water molecules leave capillaries to hydrate cells, they encounter areas of low water/high toxin concentrations and are osmotically compelled to stay there, almost as if to dilute the toxins.

If there is not enough water in the body to flush out toxins, whatever water is available stays in the connective tissues. Therefore, if the amount of pure water ingested is not sufficient to maintain a high enough water concentration gradient to drive in fresh water and drive out toxin-saturated water, waste water simply builds up in the tissues. This phenomenon is yet another manifestation of a water-deprived body desperately holding onto all the water it can.

Finally, fresh water molecules from the capillaries are accompanied by oxygen and nutrients intended to supply each cell's nutritional requirements. The stagnant build-up of water in the tissues prevents the influx of water and nutrients into the cells. Therefore, cells are left in a state of subclinical dehydration, reduced oxygenation, and nutritional deficiency.

A sedentary lifestyle is another significant factor that contributes to edema but is often overlooked by conventional medicine. The muscle movement that occurs during exercise helps move the fluids trapped in connective tissue into lymph channels, where they are returned to general circulation. Toxins then are excreted by the most appropriate means. Sedentary habits fail to provide the tissue-cleansing benefits of muscle-driven fluid movement. Thus, toxins continue to build up in the tissue, and whatever water is available is held there by osmotic attraction.

If toxic build-up within connective tissues is identified as a cause for edema, it is imperative to engage in regular exercise and flush the system thoroughly throughout the day with pure water. Such a process allows fresh water molecules and nutrients from the capillaries to traverse the connective tissue unimpeded and efficiently enter cells, giving rise to optimal hydration and nourishment. This approach resolves subclinical dehydration and associated edema.

Obesity

Obesity is a complex disorder involving issues of culturally conditioned lifestyle choices and also may include psychological issues affecting a person's emotional relationship to food. Water can be used as a significant component of an integrative regimen to address weight problems. Increased water intake is beneficial because it
— helps to control appetite,
— participates in the biochemical processes that metabolize fat,
— alleviates fluid retention and edema by easing the body's desperate need to retain water,
— flushes out toxins residing in fat tissue and releases them into the bloodstream when fat is metabolized, and

— improves metabolic activity of cells as a cofactor in energy metabolism processes.

Many people, even those who are not obese, misread body signals. Signals indicating thirst often are mistaken for signals indicating hunger. As a result, people continually eat food that their bodies don't need and fail to drink the water their bodies do need. The results are increased fat deposits and unresolved tissue thirst.

In addition to nutritional counseling and psychotherapy focused on eliminating the use of food as an emotional crutch, pure water should be a pillar of a well-designed, professionally supervised weight-management program.

Cancer

As unbelievable as it may seen to some readers, there is growing evidence that drinking pure water may reduce the risk for some forms of cancer. On deeper reflection, the relationship between hydration and malignancy becomes more apparent. Water is the carrier that removes many carcinogenic toxins from the body. Increasing water intake decreases the concentration of those toxins and hastens their removal from tissues. In addition, all body functions used to prevent and control malignant tendencies are supported in their functioning by optimal hydration.

To ward off cancer, white blood cells of the immune system scan cell membrane surface antigens to detect signs that they might turn malignant. Special enzyme complexes within the nucleus scan DNA strands to detect aberrations and subsequently make corrections in the DNA code sequence to prevent errors that disrupt healthy cell functioning. These and other routine anticancer protective processes require optimal hydration throughout the body and at the cellular level to be fully operative. Let's explore some examples in the recent scientific literature that demonstrate water's beneficial effects at preventing cancer.

Animal studies have shown that increased frequency of urination is inversely associated with carcinogen levels in the urinary tract. In other words, the more urine an animal produces, the lower the concentration of cancer-causing chemicals in contact with urinary tract tissues. To study this phenomenon in humans, researchers at the Department of Nutrition, Harvard School of Public Health, examined the relationship between total fluid intake and the risk of bladder cancer during a 10-year period, among 47,909 participants in the prospective Health Professionals Follow-up Study. Among men, "total daily fluid intake was inversely associated with the risk of bladder cancer." The consumption of water contributed to a lower relative risk than consumption of other fluids. (Michaud)

A hospital-based, case-control study was conducted in Taiwan to determine the relationship between water intake and colorectal cancer. "A strong inverse dose-response relation between increased water intake and rectal cancer was found among men after adjustment for other risk factors." (Tang)

These studies are beginning to uncover the important and previously unacknowledged connection between hydration and cancer. As rates of malignancy rise in Western civilization, it would be unwise to ignore what is being revealed.

Endless Applications

We heartily urge professionals and the public to explore the full potential of water therapy. Dr. Batmanghelidj's books are a good place to start. We have only just begun to discover the applications of water for the prevention and treatment of illness. Confirmatory scientific evidence is building rapidly. In the future, pure water will be regarded as the safest, most cost-effective, and most natural tool for preventive medicine and healing.

water

The Foundation of Youth, Health, and Beauty

References

A'o, LKK. *Don't Drink the Water*. Kali Press, 1998.

Anderson SD, Holzer K. Exercise-induced asthma: is it the right diagnosis in elite athletes? *J Allergy Clin Immunol*, 2000;106(3):419-28.

Batmanghelidj F. A new and natural method of treatment of peptic ulcer disease. *J Clin Gastroenterol* 1983;5(3):203-5.

Batmanghelidj F. *ABCs of Asthma, Allergies and Lupus*. Global Health Solutions, Inc., 2000.

Batmanghelidj F. Pain: a need for paradigm change. *Anticancer Res*, 1987; 7(5B):971-89.

Batmanghelidj F. *Your Body's Many Cries for Water*. Global Health Solutions, Inc., 1997.

Berne RM, Levy MN. *Principles of Physiology*, 3rd Edition, Mosby, Inc., 2000.

Bird PJ. Fluid needs winter and summer. University of Florida, Dept. of Health and Human Performance, 1999.

Borgnia M, et al. Cellular and molecular biology of the aquaporin water channels. *Ann Rev Biochem*, 1999;68:425-58.

Bunkin AF, Pershin SM . Influence of water cluster structure on crystallization of lysozyme from aqueous solution. *Physics of Vibrations* 2002; 10(3): 128-33.

Burke LM, Nutrition for post-exercise recovery. *Aust J Sci Med Sport*, 1997;29(1):3-10.

Carter JE, Gisolfi CV. Fluid replacement during and after exercise in the heat. *Med Sci Sports Exerc*, 1989;21(5):532-9.

Champe P, Harvey R. *Lippincott's Illustrated Reviews: Biochemistry*, 2nd ed. J. B. Lippincott Company, 1994.

Chan J, et al. Water, other fluids, and fatal coronary heart disease: the Adventist Health Study. *Am J Epidemiol*, 2002;155(9):827-33.

Chaplin M, School of Applied Sciences, South Bank University, UK.

Chebotarev AN. Study of the effects of Penta water at the cytogenetic level. Medical-Genetic evaluation of food products, Conference, Moscow, May 27-29, 2003.

Collins RD. Differential Diagnosis in Primary Care, 2nd Ed., J. B. Lippincott Company, 1987.

de Simone G, et al. Relation of blood viscosity to demographic and physiologic variables and to cardiovascular risk factors in apparently normal adults. *Circulation*, 1990;81(1):107-17.

Echevarria M, Illundain AA. Aquaporins. *J Physiol Biochem*, 1998;54(2):107-18x.

Erikssen G, et al. Haematocrit: a predictor of cardiovascular mortality? *J Intern Med*, 1993;234(5):493-9.

Garrow JS, et al, eds. *Human Nutrition and Dietetics*, 10th Ed. Churchill Livingstone, 2000.

Kannel WB, McGee DL. Update on some epidemiologic features of intermittent claudication: the Framingham Study. *J Am Geriatr Soc*, 1985;33(1):13-8.

Kelly GS. Sports nutrition. In Pizzorno J and Murray M, eds., *Textbook of Natural Medicine*, 2nd ed,. Churchill Livingstone, 1999.

King LS, Agre P. Pathophysiology of the aquaporin water channels. *Annual Rev Physiol*, 1996;58:619-48.

Kjaer A, et al. Dehydration stimulates hypothalamic gene expression of histamine synthesis enzyme: importance for neuroendocrine regulation of vasopressin and oxytocin secretion. *Endocrinology*, 1995;136(5):2189-97.

Koenig W, Ernst E. The possible role of hemorheology in atherothrombogenesis. *Atherosclerosis*, 1992;94(2-3):93-107.

Lamb DR, Brodowicz GR. Optimal use of fluids of varying formulations to minimise exercise-induced disturbances in homeostasis. *Sports Med* 1986;3(4):247-74.

Lee AJ, et al. Blood viscosity and elevated carotid intima-media thickness in men and women: the Edinburgh Artery Study. *Circulation*, 1998;97(15):1467-73.

Lowe GD, et al. Blood viscosity and risk of cardiovascular events: the Edinburgh Artery Study. *Br J Haematol*, 1997;96(1):168-73.

Lowe GD, et al. Relation between extent of coronary artery disease and blood viscosity. *Br Med J*, 1980;280(6215):673-4.

Ma T, Verkman AS. Aquaporin water channels in gastrointestinal physiology. *J Physiol*, 1999;517 (Pt 2):317-26.

Maughan RJ, Noakes TD. Fluid replacement and exercise stress. A brief review of studies on fluid replacement and some guidelines for the athlete. *Sports Med*, 1991;12(1):16-31.

Maughan RJ, et al. Effects of ingested fluids on exercise capacity and on cardiovascular and metabolic responses to prolonged exercise in man. *Exp Physiol*, 1996;81(5):847-59.

Medrala W, et al. Pathogenesis of exercise induced asthma. *Pol Merkuriusz Lek* 2001;11(63):203-5.

Michaud DS, et al. Fluid intake and the risk of bladder cancer in men. *N Engl J Med*,1999;340(18):1390-7.

Murray M. *Encyclopedia of Nutritional Supplements*. Prima Publishing, 1996.

Neufer PD, et al. Effects of exercise and carbohydrate composition on gastric emptying. *Med Sci Sports Exerc,* 1986;18(6):658-62.

Phillips PA, et al. Reduced thirst after water deprivation in healthy elderly men. *N Engl J Med,* 1984;311(12):753-9.

Pizzorno J, Murray M, eds. *Textbook of Natural Medicine,* 2nd ed,. Churchill Livingstone, 1999.

Rehrer NJ, et al. Exercise and training effects on gastric emptying of carbohydrate beverages. *Med Sci Sports Exerc,* 1989;21(5):540-9.

Rehrer NJ, et al. Gastric emptying with repeated drinking during running and bicycling. *Int J Sports Med,* 1990;11(3):238-43.

Resch KL, et al. Can rheologic variables be of prognostic relevance in arteriosclerotic diseases? *Angiology,* 1991;42(12):963-70.

Rothfeder J. *Every Drop for Sale: Our Desperate Battle for Water in a World About to Run Out.* Penguin Putnam, 2001.

Schwartz J, et al, Drinking water turbidity and gastrointestinal illness in the elderly of Phillips PA. Reduced thirst after water deprivation in healthy elderly men. *N Engl J Med* 1984 Sep 20;311(12):753-9.

Streeten D. Bell D. Circulation blood volume in chronic fatigue syndrome. *Journal of CFS,* 1998;4(1):3.

Tang R, et al. Physical activity, water intake and risk of colorectal cancer in Taiwan: a hospital-based case-control study. *Int J Cancer,* 1999;82(4):484-9.

Terrados N, Maughan RJ. Exercise in the heat: strategies to minimize the adverse effects on performance. *J Sports Sci,* 1995;13 Spec No:S55-62.

Turovetsky V. Cell survivability and intracellular pH study. [In preparation for publication].

Venero JL, et al. Aquaporins in the central nervous system. *Prog Neurobiol,* 2001;63(3):321-36.

Verkman AS, Mitra AK. Structure and function of aquaporin water channels. *Am J Physiol Renal Physiol,* 2000;278(1):F13-28.

Verkman AS, et al. Aquaporin water channels and lung physiology. *Am J Physiol Lung Cell Mol Physiol,* 2000;278(5):L867-79.

Von Os CH, et al. Physiological relevance of aquaporins: luxury or necessity? *Eur J Physiol,* 2000;440:513-20.

Watterson JG. The role of water in cell architecture. *Mol Cell Biochem,* 1988;79(2):101-5.

Yamamoto T, Sasaki S. Aquaporins in the kidney: emerging new aspects. *Kidney Int,* 1998;54(4):1041-51.